MW00580981

Pharmacy Technician Certification

Review *and* Practice Exam

SECOND EDITION

LINDA FRED, R.PH.

DIRECTOR OF INPATIENT PHARMACY SERVICES
CARLE FOUNDATION HOSPITAL

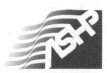

American Society of Health-System Pharmacists®
Bethesda, Maryland

Any correspondence regarding this publication should be sent to the publisher, American Society of Health-System Pharmacists, 7272 Wisconsin Avenue, Bethesda, MD 20814, attn: Special Publishing. Produced in conjunction with the ASHP Publications Production Center.

The information presented herein reflects the opinions of the contributors and reviewers. It should not be interpreted as an official policy of ASHP or as an endorsement of any product.

This review book is not sponsored or endorsed by the Pharmacy Technician Certification Board (PTCB). Although every effort has been made on behalf of the authors, editor, and publisher to provide an extensive review, comprehension of the material included in this text and the practice exam does not guarantee successful completion of the PTCB national certification examination or any other examination. The practice exam represents the opinions of the authors and editors of this work and has not been field-tested or reviewed by PTCB.

The authors, editor, and publisher of this work have made a conscientious effort to provide the reader with accurate and up to-date information, but the nature of the information is evolving, and may be subject to change due to the dynamic nature of drug information and drug distribution systems. This information should be used solely in preparation for the certification exam or other academic purposes. No information contained in this text should be used to provide patient care.

Acquisitions Editor: Cynthia Reilly

Editorial Project Manager: Dana Battaglia

Production Manager: Johnna Hershey

Page composition: David Wade

Contents

Preface

Pharmacy Technician Certification Review and Practice Exam, second edition, is a self-study guide that is designed as a companion book to the *Manual for Pharmacy Technicians,* third edition. The objective of this book is to assist technicians who are preparing to take the Pharmacy Technician Certification Examination offered through the Pharmacy Technician Certification Board (PTCB) or other pharmacy technician examinations.

The first three sections are designed to cover the knowledge and skills areas described by the PTCB. Additional sections provide helpful study and test-taking strategies, a review of pharmacy math, information on commonly prescribed medications, and a practice exam. The book is only one tool to be used in preparation for the certification exam and is not intended to be used as the sole preparation guide for the certification exam.

Some activities are mastered primarily through the work experience of the individual and cannot be adequately explained through didactic material. The book should be used in conjunction with the *Manual for Pharmacy Technicians,* third edition, other study aids recommended in the PTCB candidate handbook, and job experience.

Linda Fred, Editor
2004

Contributors

ASHP gratefully acknowledges the following individuals for their contribution to the *Manual for Pharmacy Technicians,* third edition, which served as the foundation for this publication.

Bonnie S. Bachenheimer, Pharm.D.
Drug Information Clinical Specialist
Advocate Lutheran General Hospital
Park Ridge, Illinois

Karen E. Bertch, Pharm.D., FCCP
Director, Pharmacy Services, Product Planning,
Premier, Incorporated
Oak Brook, Illinois
Per Diem Clinical Pharmacist
Coram Healthcare
Mt. Prospect, Illinois

Linda Y. Fred, R.Ph.
Director of Inpatient Pharmacy Services
Carle Foundation Hospital
Urbana, Illinois

Alice J.A. Gardner, Ph.D.
Assistant Professor of Pharmacology and Toxicology
Department of Pharmaceutical Sciences
Massachusetts College of Pharmacy & Health Sciences
School of Pharmacy-Worcester
Worcester, Massachusetts

Douglas C. Higgins, R.Ph.
Doug's Pharmacy
Paxton, Illinois

Rebecca Kentzel, CPhT
Manager of Project Management Office
OSF Healthcare System
Mackinaw, Illinois

Jacqueline Z. Kessler, M.S., R.Ph., FASHP
Clinical Specialist
Advocate Lutheran General Hospital
Park Ridge, Illinois

Tanya C. Knight-Klimas, Pharm.D., CGP, FASCP
Clinical Assistant Professor of Pharmacy
Temple University School of Pharmacy
Clinical Geriatric Pharmacist
Living Independently For Elders (LIFE)
Saint Agnes Medical Center
Philadelphia, PA

continued

Connie Larson, Pharm.D.
Medication Safety Officer
Assistant Director, Safety and Quality
Hospital Pharmacy Services
University of Illinois Medical Center at Chicago
Chicago, Illinois

Richard K. Lewis, Pharm.D., MBA
Continuing Education Administrator
ProCE, Incorporated

Steven Lundquist, Pharm.D.
Clinical Director
Cardinal Health
Pharmacy Management
Marco Island, Florida

Scott M. Mark, Pharm.D., M.S., M.Ed., CHE, FASHP
Director of Pharmacy
Children's National Medical Center
Washington, District of Columbia

Jerrod Milton, BScPharm
Adjunct Assistant Clinical Professor
University of Colorado Health Sciences Center,
School of Pharmacy
Director, Pharmacy Services
The Children's Hospital
Denver, Colorado

Diane F. Pacitti, Ph.D., R.Ph.
Assistant Professor of Pharmaceutical Sciences
Massachusetts College of Pharmacy and Health Sciences
Worcester, Massachusetts

Michele F. Shepherd, Pharm.D., M.S., FASHP, BCPS
Clinical Specialist
Department of Medical Education
Abbott Northwestern Hospital
Minneapolis, Minnesota

Sheri Stensland, Pharm.D.
Assistant Professor of Pharmacy Practice
Shared Faculty for Walgreens
Midwestern University Chicago College of Pharmacy
Downers Grove, Illinois

Gerald A. Storm, R.Ph.
Director of Pharmacy
OSF-Saint Francis Medical Center
Peoria, Illinois

Philip R. Torf, R.Ph., J.D.
Attorney-at-Law
Torf Law Firm
Northbrook, Illinois
Administrator
Institute for Pharmacy Law
Northbrook, Illinois

Assisting the Pharmacist

Medication Orders and Prescriptions Defined

Typically, the term *medication order* refers to a written request on a physician's order form or a transcribed verbal or telephone order in an inpatient setting. This order becomes part of the patient's medical record. The term *prescription* refers to a medication order on a prescription blank to be filled in an outpatient or ambulatory care setting. The two serve essentially the same purpose. They both represent a means of communication for the prescriber to give instruction to the dispenser of the medication or to those who will be administering the medication.

Pharmacy Terms and Abbreviations

Pharmacy personnel use a number of terms in their work. An understanding of these terms helps a technician to be efficient and capable.

Some of these terms define classifications of drugs. For example, technicians must be able to differentiate between *generic* and *brand name* drugs. A generic name describes a unique chemical entity and can be applied to that entity regardless of its manufacturer. A brand name is trademarked by a manufacturer to identify its particular "brand" of that chemical entity. For example, Ancef® is a brand name product of the generic entity cefazolin.

Another pair of terms used to categorize drugs is *legend* and *over-the-counter*. A legend drug, also called a prescription drug, is one that may not be dispensed to the public except on the order of a physician or other licensed prescriber. The term comes from the federal legend that appears on the packaging: "Federal law prohibits dispensing this medication without a prescription." Over-the-counter medications may be sold to the public without a prescription as long as they are properly labeled for home use.

One last term, *formulary*, is used in slightly different ways in institutional and retail settings. A formulary is a listing of approved drugs available for use. In a hospital, it refers to the drugs that are stocked by the pharmacy and approved for use in the facility. In the retail setting, the term is generally applied to an approved drug list associated with a particular benefit plan.

Pharmacy abbreviations are commonly used as a kind of shorthand in prescriptions and medication orders to convey information about directions for use. The abbreviations are then "translated" on the prescription

Learning Objectives

After completing this chapter, the technician should be able to

1. Define the terms *medication order* and *prescription* and list the common means by which they are received by the pharmacy.

2. Define commonly used pharmacy terms and abbreviations used in medication orders and prescriptions.

3. List the required elements on a prescription or medication order.

4. Describe the steps required for proper prescription and medication order processing.

5. Explain good compounding practices and aseptic technique.

6. List and describe the equipment used in both sterile and nonsterile compounding.

7. Describe the types of questions that may be answered by a pharmacy technician.

8. List common references found in many pharmacies and what information might be found in each.

9. Describe charging mechanisms used in inpatient and outpatient settings.

10. Describe how prescriptions are transferred between pharmacies.

label. **Table 1-1** lists many commonly used pharmacy abbreviations.

The abbreviations for time and frequency of medication administration come from Latin phrases. Other commonly used abbreviations include those for routes of administration and those that designate units of measure. Lowercase Roman numerals are often used to denote a quantity, such as a number of tablets (i = one; ii = two). (See Chapter 5 of *Manual for Pharmacy Technicians* for a review of Roman numerals.)

Another subset of abbreviations is called *x-Substitutions* and includes the well-known and widely recognized *Rx* symbol, meaning *prescription*. Other common x-substitutions are *dx* for *diagnosis* and *sx* for *symptoms*.

Abbreviations in medical records and in prescriptions are thought to be contributing factors in some medical errors. One important example is the use of the letter *U* to abbreviate units. Because a *U* might be misread as a zero if sloppily written—and could therefore result in a tenfold dosing error—the Institute for Safe Medication Practices recommends that it never be used as an abbreviation in prescriptions or medication orders; the word *units* should always be written out in its entirety. Other abbreviations that some consider unsafe are *q.d., q.i.d.,* and *q.o.d.*, which may be indistinguishable from each other if legibility is poor. These three abbreviations have been included in the chapter because they are still widely used.

Receiving and Processing Medication Orders in a Hospital

Medication orders come to the hospital pharmacy in various ways. They can be delivered to the pharmacy or one of its satellites in person or via some mechanical method, such as fax transmission or a pneumatic tube system. Orders may also be telephoned to the pharmacy by either the prescriber or an intermediary, such as a nurse. There are some legal restrictions on who may telephone in an order or a prescription and who may receive that information in the pharmacy—particularly when controlled substances are involved.

Ideally, every medication order should contain the following elements:

- Patient name, hospital identification number, and room/bed location
- Generic drug name (using generic drug names is recommended, and many institutions have policies to this effect)

- Brand drug name (if a specific product is required)
- Route of administration (with some orders, the site of administration should also be included)
- Dosage form
- Dose/strength
- Frequency and duration of administration (if duration is pertinent—may be open-ended)
- Rate and time of administration, if applicable
- Indication for use of the medication
- Other instructions for the person administering the medication, such as whether it should be given with food or on an empty stomach
- Prescriber's name/signature and credentials (some hospitals require a printed name, physician number, or pager number in addition to the signature to assist with identification)
- Signature and credentials of person writing the order if other than prescriber
- Date and time of the order

When a new order is received, the first step is to ensure that the order is clear and complete. If information is missing—for example, the room number for the patient, the technician may be able to clarify the order without pharmacist intervention. Some clarifications, however, should involve the pharmacist. (See the discussion of which questions can be handled by a technician later in this chapter.)

Once orders are deemed clear and complete, they must be prioritized so that the most urgent orders are filled first. Prioritizing orders means comparing the urgency of new orders with the urgency of all the orders requiring attention. This ensures that those orders needed the most will be processed first. Technicians can prioritize orders by evaluating the route, time of administration, type of drug, intended use of the drug, and patient-specific circumstances.

A number of steps are involved in processing an order in the computer. First, the patient must be positively identified to avoid dispensing medication for the wrong patient. Second, the order is typically compared with the patient's existing medication profile, or a new profile is created for the patient. Then, the technician takes a number of order entry steps to update the patient's medication profile.

TABLE 1-1. COMMONLY USED PHARMACY ABBREVIATIONS

Abbreviation	Meaning	Latin Phrase	Abbreviation	Meaning	Latin Phrase
a	before	*ante*	OS	left eye	
a.c.	before meals	*ante cibum*	OTC	over-the-counter	
ad lib	as desired	*ad libitum*	OU	both eyes	
AD	right ear		oz	ounce	
AS	left ear		p	post	*post*
AU	both ears		p.c.	after meals	*post cibum*
b.i.d.	twice a day	*bis in die*	p.o.	by mouth	*per os*
bx	biopsy		pr	per rectum	
c	with		p.r.n.	as needed	*pro re nata*
cc	cubic centimeter		pt	pint	
dr	dram		q.	every	*quaque*
dx	diagnosis		q.a.m.	every morning	
fx	fracture		q.d.	every day	*quaque die*
g	gram		q.h.	every hour	*quaque hora*
gr	grain		q2h, q3h, etc.	every 2 hours, etc.	
gtt	drop		q.i.d.	four times a day	*quarter in die*
h	hour		q.o.d.	every other day	
hr	hour		qt	quart	
h.s.	at bedtime	*hora somni*	rx, Rx	prescription	
hx	history		s	without	
ID	intradermal(ly)		sc, S.C., s.q., subq	subcutaneous	
IM	intramuscular(ly)		ss	one half	
IU	international unit		stat	immediately	
IV	intravenous(ly)		supp	suppository	
IVPB	IV piggyback		sx	symptoms	
kg	kilogram		T, Tbsp	tablespoon	
L	liter		t, tsp	teaspoon	
lb	pound		t.i.d.	three times a day	*ter in die*
mcg	microgram		T.O.	telephone order	
mEq	milliequivalent		tr	tincture	
mg	milligram		tx	treatment	
ml	milliliter		ung	ointment	
OD	right eye		VO	verbal order	

The following step-by-step process outlines a fairly typical medication order entry process. Systems vary somewhat, however, and this is simply an example of what the process flow might look like.

1. Enter the patient's name or medical record number and verify them to ensure that the correct patient record has been chosen.

2. Compare the order with the patient profile in detail to look for duplications or other possible problems or to create the patient profile. Check for general appropriateness of the order; it should make sense in regard to patient profile information, such as the patient's age, allergies, and drugs currently being taken. The following information is appropriately found in the hospital pharmacy's patient profile, although system capabilities may limit access to some components:

   - Patient name and identification number
   - Date of birth, or age
   - Sex
   - Height and weight
   - Certain lab values, such as creatinine clearance
   - Admitting and secondary diagnoses (including pregnancy and lactation status)
   - Name of parent or guardian, if applicable
   - Room and bed number
   - Names of admitting and consulting physicians
   - Medication allergies; latex allergy; pertinent food allergies
   - Medication history (current and discontinued medications; medications from a previous admission in some instances)
   - Special considerations (e.g., foreign language, disability)
   - Clinical comments (e.g., therapeutic monitoring, counseling notes)

3. Enter the drug. Selecting the correct drug product requires a working knowledge of both brand names and generic names (although most computer systems can search for either name) and a sensible approach to interpreting orders when abbreviations are used. When in doubt about a drug name or an abbreviation, however, it is always better to clarify the order with the prescriber or the person who wrote the order. Patient safety must be protected, and it is dangerous to make assumptions when interpreting orders. Most pharmacies take special precautions to ensure accurate interpretation of prescriptions and medication orders involving look-alike and sound-alike drugs. With most pharmacy computer systems, drug products can be reviewed by scrolling through an alphabetical listing of the brand or generic names or by entering a code or mnemonic that is associated with the product name in the computer. Many computer systems alert the operator if he or she attempts to enter medications that interact with current orders, conflict with the patient's drug allergies, represent therapeutic duplications, or are nonformulary drugs. Many systems also check the dosage range and alert the pharmacist or technician if he or she enters a dose that exceeds the recommended dose for that patient. Although these alert systems help prevent errors, they are not always significant given the patient's unique situation. Therefore, the technician must consult the pharmacist when the alert is posted. Besides just choosing the "correct drug" as has been outlined in this section, some other related choices are included in this step. For example, if an intravenous (IV) medication is being entered, it might be necessary to choose the correct diluent into which the drug is to be mixed. Another decision involved in choosing the correct drug is the choice of the package type and size—bulk or unit dose, 15 gram tube or 30 gram tube, 100 ml bottle or 150 ml bottle.

4. Verify the dose to ensure that the correct amount has been entered.

5. Enter the administration schedule. In institutions, standard medication administration times are generally set. These schedules are usually based on therapeutic issues or nursing efficiency or are designed to coordinate services, such as laboratory blood draws or therapy schedules. Standard administration schedules and protocols are usually agreed upon by pharmacy, nursing, and the hospital's medical staff. Many pharmacies have a written document, such as a policy, that staff can refer to when the appropriate administration time is unclear.

6.	Enter any comments in the *clinical comments* field. The prescriber's directions for proper use of the medications must be conveyed clearly and accurately. Additional instructions for the caregiver are often entered into the pharmacy information system for presentation on one of the many documents printed from the profile (or for the nurses' use in an electronic system) or simply as additional information for the pharmacists' use at a later time. These special instructions might include storage information, such as the need to refrigerate, or special instructions, such as for chemotherapy drugs. Another example would be physician-specified parameters for use, such as "hold if systolic BP less than 100 mm Hg" or "repeat in one hour if ineffective." These types of instructions would typically be displayed on the medication administration record (MAR) and also on the medication label.

7.	Verify the prescriber name.

8.	Fill and label the medication. Once the computer entry has been completed and labeling materials generated, the medication order must be filled with the correct quantity of the correct drug. During this step, the technician should carefully review the label against the order and the product to be used to make sure the correct product has been chosen. This is the final opportunity for the pharmacy to catch an error before dispensing to a patient care area. The medication order is then filled and left for the pharmacist to check. With few exceptions, this pharmacist check is legally required before dispensing any drug to a patient care area.

Receiving and Processing Prescriptions in an Outpatient Pharmacy

In the past, prescriptions were presented to the pharmacy by the patient after having been written by the prescribing physician on a prescription blank. Now, however, prescriptions can come in to the pharmacy by a number of other means. Many prescriptions are telephoned in from the prescriber's office. Other means of communication include facsimile and electronic transmission. Many pharmacies also accept refill requests over the Internet through a pharmacy Web page.

Obtaining payer information is an important step in receiving a prescription in the outpatient setting. This information is used for a number of purposes, including establishing the primary payer for the prescription, the patient's portion of the reimbursement (copay), and in some instances the drug formulary.

Reviewing a prescription for clarity and completeness is similar in the outpatient and the inpatient setting. The following prescription elements are typically present:

■	Patient name

■	Patient home address

■	Date the prescription was written

■	Drug name—either generic or brand

■	Drug strength and dose to be administered

■	Directions for use, including route of administration, frequency, and, as applicable, duration of use (some durations are open-ended)

■	Quantity to be dispensed

■	Number of refills to be allowed

■	Substitution authority or refusal

■	Signature and credentials of the prescriber and Drug Enforcement Agency (DEA) number, if required

■	Reason for use, or indication (not generally required)

In an ambulatory practice, some special clarity and completeness issues must be considered. When the prescriber uses "Dispense As Written," or DAW, on the prescription blank, the brand name drug written on the prescription must be dispensed. Another outpatient issue is prescription forgeries, particularly for controlled substances.

Assessing Order Authenticity

Screening prescriptions, particularly those for controlled substances, for potential forgeries is part of routine prescription processing. The technician should screen prescriptions for anything that looks unusual, such as a dispense quantity in excess of normal quantities or an unusual or unrecognizable signature. Any suspicious prescription should be discreetly presented to the pharmacist for further evaluation.

Prescription forgeries often take one of two forms: (1) erasure or overwriting of the strength or dispensing quantity of the drug (e.g., changing a 3 to an 8), and

(2) theft of preprinted prescription pads that may result in legitimate-looking prescriptions.

One thing a technician can do to help prevent prescription forgery is determine whether a DEA number on a controlled substance prescription is valid. A valid DEA number consists of two letters and seven numbers, such as "BB 1 1 9 7 9 6 7." If the holder of the DEA number is a registrant, such as a physician or pharmacy, the first letter is an "A" or "B." If the holder of the DEA number is a mid-level practitioner, such as a qualified nurse practitioner, the first letter is an "M." The second letter is related to the registrant's name. In the case of a physician, it is the first letter of his or her last name.

The seven numbers are also used to determine a legitimate DEA number. The odd group—the 1st, 3rd, and 5th numbers in the sequence, and the even group—the 2nd, 4th, and 6th numbers—are added in the following manner so that the sum relates to the 7th number:

BB 1 1 9 7 9 6 7

Odd Group $1 + 9 + 9 = 19$

Even Group $1 + 7 + 6 = 14$

Sum of odd (19) and 2 × even group (14 × 2) =
$19 + 28 = 47$

The last digit of this odd/even group sum is the same as the last digit of the DEA number.

Prioritization of prescription processing in the outpatient pharmacy is generally an issue of customer service rather than patient care.

Prescription processing includes many of the same steps as medication order processing in the inpatient setting:

- Identifying the patient: It is important to make sure that prescriptions are filled for and dispensed to the correct patient. Proper attention needs to be paid to similar or identical names to make sure the medication is profiled on the right patient profile. Another important concern for the outpatient staff at this stage is to ensure that there is no forgery and that the individuals obtaining controlled substances are lawfully entitled to do so.

- Creating, maintaining, and reviewing patient profiles: A number of pieces of information are typically collected in the patient profile—some according to law (which varies from state to state) and some for efficiency and convenience purposes for both the pharmacy and the patient. These pieces of information include the following:

  - Patient's name and identification number
  - Age or date of birth
  - Home address and telephone number
  - Allergies
  - Principle diagnoses of patient
  - Primary health care providers for patient
  - Third-party payer(s) and other billing information
  - Over-the-counter medications and herbal supplements used by the patient
  - Prescription and refill history of the patient
  - Patient preferences (e.g., child-resistant packaging waiver, preference for receiving prescriptions by mail)

Once the patient's profile is located or created and the existing information verified, selecting the appropriate drug product is the next step in the order entry process. Most outpatient computer systems, like inpatient systems, allow drug product choice by typing in a mnemonic or by accessing an alphabetical listing of some sort. These are the typical prescription processing steps:

1. Enter the patient's medical record number or name and verify them. This safety step ensures that the drug is dispensed to the correct patient.

2. Enter or verify existing third-party billing information to ensure correct billing and copayment.

3. Compare the order with the patient profile in detail to identify duplications or other concerns.

4. Enter the prescription. A variety of information must be entered into the computer at this point, and systems vary as to the order in which it is entered. The following are required elements:

- Physician's name
- Directions for use, including special comments
- Fill quantity
- Initials of the pharmacist checking the prescription
- Number of refills authorized

At the time of computer processing, an error message may interrupt transmission of the prescription to the third-party payer. The following are some common error messages and their meanings:

■ *Refill Too Soon*: This message deals with refill prescriptions and the elapsed time between filling prescriptions. Typically, third parties allow patients to receive a 30-day supply of medications. If the patient attempts to refill a prescription within a significantly shorter period (e.g., 15 days after the last prescription), the prescription cannot be processed without prior approval from the third-party payer.

■ *Missing/Invalid Patient ID*: This or a similar message indicates that the patient who is entered into the pharmacy computer does not appear to be enrolled in the insurance program. On receiving this message, the technician should examine the patient information entered for mistakes. Perhaps the name was misspelled, identification number mistyped, or other required information left out. Because many insurance plans use a Pharmacy Benefit Manager (PBM) to manage their pharmacy services, the prescription may need to be processed under the name of the PBM instead of the name of the third-party payer.

■ *Drug–Drug or Drug–Allergy Interaction*: Most pharmacy software will screen the patient profile for drug and allergy information. If interactions are detected, the program will alert the user. Some software will not only identify an interaction but also indicate its potential severity. A technician who receives a drug-drug or drug–allergy interaction message should alert the pharmacist to the problem.

■ *Nonformulary/Not Covered*: Many third-party payers have formularies (lists of covered drugs). This message indicates that the drug is not covered, and payment will not be made for that drug. A technician who receives this message should alert the pharmacist.

5. Fill and label the prescription. The following components must generally appear on a prescription label, whether typed or computer-generated (may vary by state):

   ■ Patient's name

   ■ Date the prescription is being filled (or refilled)

   ■ Prescriber's name

   ■ Sequential prescription number

   ■ Name of the drug (including manufacturer if filled generically)

   ■ Quantity to be dispensed

   ■ Directions for use

   ■ Number of refills remaining (or associated refill period)

Labeling includes more than just the actual prescription label. The inpatient section of this chapter noted that labeling for inpatient use is often abbreviated or in a form of shorthand. For home use, however, this practice is not acceptable. Beyond the prescription label itself, auxiliary information is often included in the form of special labels affixed to the container or drug information leaflets for patients to read at home. Instructions for home use must include the following at a minimum:

■ Administration directions (e.g., "Take," "Insert," "Apply")

■ Number of units constituting one dose and the dosage form (e.g., 2 tablets)

■ Route of administration (e.g., "by mouth," "vaginally")

■ How frequently or at what time (e.g., "twice daily," "daily at 9 a.m.")

■ Length of time to continue, if applicable (e.g., "for 10 days," "until finished")

■ Indication of purpose, if applicable (e.g., "for pain," "for blood pressure")

At the time of dispensing, the pharmacist or technician must be sure the patient fully understands how to use the medication. This is also an appropriate time to consider language barriers, such as illiteracy or a primary language other than English.

Good Compounding Practices

Chemicals for compounding are approved by the Food and Drug Administration (FDA); however, the practice of compounding is controlled by the individual state boards of pharmacy. Certain aspects of compounding and the role of the FDA were not clearly defined in federal law until, in 1997, the Food and Drug Administration Modernization Act (FDAMA) was passed. This legislation clearly defined the roles of both compounding pharmacies and the FDA. In the summer of 2002, however, the legislation was declared unconstitutional because of advertising restrictions. Nonetheless, the guidelines of the 1997 FDAMA still offer a structure for compounding pharmacists to follow until future legislation addresses the issue.

The *United States Pharmacopeia (USP 27)* offers guidelines for compounding. The following chapters of the *USP 27* review specific areas of compounding:

- Chapter 795 Pharmaceutical Compounding—Nonsterile Preparations
- Chapter 797 Pharmaceutical Compounding—Sterile Preparations
- Chapter 1075 Good Compounding Practices

The following are key areas of compounding:

1. Responsibility of the compounder
2. Compounding environment
3. Stability of compounded preparations
4. Ingredient selection
5. Compounded preparations
6. Compounding processes
7. Compounding records and documents
8. Material Safety Data Sheets (MSDS) file
9. Quality control
10. Patient counseling

Responsibility of the Compounder

The compounder is responsible for all aspects of the compounding process, including, but not limited to, appropriately trained personnel and the key areas of Chapter 795 of the *USP 27* that follow.

Compounding Environment

The compounding area should have adequate space for equipment and support materials. Controlled temperature and lighting are needed for chemicals and finished medications. The area must be kept clean for sanitary reasons and to prevent cross contamination. A sink with hot and cold running water is essential for handwashing and cleaning of equipment.

Stability of Compounded Preparations

Stability is defined in *USP 27* as "the extent to which a preparation retains, within specified limits, and throughout its period of storage and use, the same properties and characteristics that is possessed at the time of compounding."[1] (See Recommended Reading.)

Primary packaging of the finished medication is of utmost importance. The choice of container is guided by the physical and chemical characteristics of the finished medication. Considerations such as light sensitivity and the medication binding to the container are examples of concern in maximizing stability.

Beyond-use labeling should be included on all medications (expiration dates apply to manufactured products). Examples of considerations for determining beyond-use dates include whether the medication is aqueous or nonaqueous, expiration date of the ingredients used, storage temperature, references documenting the stability of the finished medication, and the *USP*.

Ingredient Selection

Sources of ingredients vary widely. USP or National Formulary (NF) chemicals are the preferred source of chemicals for compounding. Other sources may be used, but the compounder has a responsibility to be certain the chemical meets purity and safety standards. Manufactured medications are another acceptable source of ingredients. It would be inappropriate to use any chemical withdrawn from use by the FDA.

Compounded Preparations

Preparations should contain at least 90 percent, but not more than 110 percent, of the labeled active ingredient, unless more restrictive laws apply. Compounding guidelines in *USP 27* specifically address the following drug forms:

- Capsules, powders, lozenges, and tablets
- Emulsions, solutions, and suspensions
- Suppositories
- Creams, topical gels, ointments, and pastes

Compounding Processes

The goal of the compounding process is to "minimize error and maximize the prescriber's intent."[2] The following list is a sample of areas to consider in the compounding process:

- Evaluation of the appropriateness of the prescription
- Calculations of the amount of ingredients
- Identification of equipment needed to properly compound the prescription
- Proper hand cleaning and gowning
- Evaluation of the final medication for weight variation, proper mixing, and consistency

- Proper notations in the compounding log
- Appropriate labeling of the final medication

Compounding Records and Documents
The goal of record-keeping is to allow another compounder to reproduce the same formulation at a later date. Two parts of the records and documentation are the *formula,* or *formulation record,* and the *batch log,* or *compounding record.*

The formulation record is a file of compounded preparations, much like a recipe. It would include chemicals in the formula, equipment needed to prepare the formula, and mixing instructions for preparing the formula.

The compounding record is the log (or record) of an actual batch being prepared. It would include manufacturers and lot numbers of chemicals used, the date of preparation, an internal identification number (commonly called lot number), a beyond-use date, and any other pertinent information regarding the preparation.

MSDS File
MSDS should be readily accessible to all employees.

Quality Control
Quality control is a final check on the preparation to ensure safety and quality of the preparation. The compounder should evaluate the finished preparation both physically and by reviewing the compounding procedure to be certain the preparation is accurate. Discrepancies should be noted and evaluated to determine if the preparation is acceptable.

Patient Counseling
With any prescription, the patient should be counseled on the correct use of the medication. Compounded medications are often different in method of use or the type of dispensing container used, so special care should be taken to be certain the patient understands the proper use of the medication.

Equipment Used in Nonsterile Compounding
Compounding requires specialized equipment to obtain the best quality medications. An electronic balance is commonly used for speed and accuracy of measurement (see **Figure 1-1**).

Mortars and pestles are used to crush, grind, and blend various ingredients. The mortar is a deep bowl, and the pestle is a club-shaped tool that when stamped or pounded vertically into the well of the mortar causes the contents of the mortar to become pulverized (see **Figure 1-2**). Mixing is usually achieved by moving the pestle in a circular motion in the mortar. Mortars are available in a variety of materials and sizes. Glass, porcelain, ceramic, and Wedgwood™ are commonly used. Wedgwood™ offers a rough surface to allow grinding and reduction of particle size but is very difficult to clean and thus prevent cross contamination of preparations. Glass and porcelain offer smooth, easily cleaned surfaces.

Ointment mills are commonly found in compounding pharmacies. Most have three rollers with small, adjustable spaces between the rollers (see **Figure 1-3**). When preparations pass through the rollers, particle size is reduced.

Parenteral Drug Administration
Medications can be administered to patients in numerous ways. Medications not given to patients by mouth (enterally) are referred to as *parenterally* adminis-

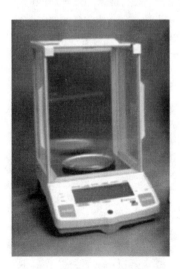

Figure 1-1. Electronic balance

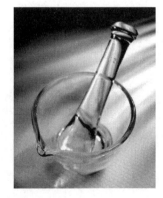

Figure 1-2. Mortar and pestle

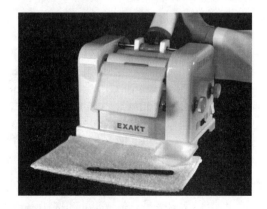

Figure 1-3. Ointment mill

tered. Parenteral administrations can include intravenous (IV), intramuscular (IM), and subcutaneous (SQ), or below the skin. IV solutions are commonly administered to patients as a means of replacing body fluids and as a vehicle for introducing drugs into the body. Medications are not beneficial to the patient until they reach the blood and are distributed to the body. IV medications are introduced directly into the blood and therefore have the most rapid onset of action. IV medications, therefore, have many benefits over oral medications, which have to be absorbed from the gastrointestinal tract, or IM medications, which have to be absorbed through the muscle mass. IV medications can be given to patients who are unconscious, uncooperative, nauseated, vomiting, or otherwise unable to take medications orally. Direct administration of IV medications into the blood also provides a predictable rate of administration. Certainly, IV medications have disadvantages, such as the risk of infection, the pain of the injection, and the immediate effect of the administration in the event of an error. Some medications are not suitable for IV administration because of their stability or absorptive properties.

Special training is required for personnel who prepare and administer sterile IV solutions. The process of preparing IV products using preset steps to ensure a sterile final product is known as *aseptic technique*. Basic aseptic technique should be used when handling parenteral dosage forms, as well as irrigations and ophthalmics (see Chapter 7 of the *Manual for Pharmacy Technicians*, Medication Dosage Forms and Routes of Administration).

Risks of IV Therapy

IV therapy offers a rapid, direct means of administering many life-saving drugs and fluids. A high percentage of IV therapy is administered without any problems, but there are some risks:

- *Infection*—Infections can result if a product contaminated with bacteria is infused into a patient. Because the IV bypasses the body's normal barrier system, bacteria reach the bloodstream directly. Bacteria can be introduced into products during preparation, administration, and production, through improper storage. The rate of infection or sepsis due to contaminated infusions has steadily decreased since health care practitioners and product manufacturers have implemented training and quality assurance programs. Despite these efforts, human touch

contamination continues to be the most common source of IV-related contamination.

- *Air embolus*—The incidence of an air embolus is low because many solutions are administered using infusion pumps equipped with an alarm, called an *air-in-line alarm*, that sounds when air is in the IV line. Solutions infused by gravity do not need alarms because the infusion automatically stops when there is no more fluid for gravity to push through the IV line. Even when a bag runs dry, large amounts of air are not infused. In adults, 150 or 200 ml of air given quickly through an IV can result in harm. Infants and pediatric patients are adversely affected by a much lower amount of air.[3] Filters are available on some IV sets, and they also stop air bubbles and add another measure of safety.

- *Bleeding*—IV therapy may cause bleeding. When the IV catheter is removed, bleeding may occur around the catheter site. If the patient has a condition that results in prolonged bleeding time, extra care and caution should be used, especially when removing the catheter.

- *Allergic reaction*—When a patient has an allergic reaction to a substance given parenterally, the reaction is usually more severe than if the same substance were given by another route (e.g., by mouth, topically, or rectally). One reason for this is that substances given parenterally cannot be retrieved like substances given by other routes. For example, substances administered topically can easily be washed off, those given orally can be retrieved by inducing vomiting or by pumping the stomach, and those given rectally can be flushed out using an enema. When a drug that has caused allergic reactions in a large number of patients is given intravenously, the patient should be monitored closely. If the likelihood of an allergic reaction is especially high, a test dose (a small amount of the drug) may be given to see how the patient reacts.

- *Incompatibilities*—Some drugs are incompatible with other drugs, containers, or solutions. If an incompatibility exists, the drug may precipitate, be inactivated, or adhere to the container. These undesirable outcomes may be difficult to detect with the naked eye. A visual inspection of the final product should always be performed to observe any cloudiness, coring, or signs of irregularity. Solutions with known or detectable incompatibilities should not be administered to patients.

- *Extravasation*—Extravasation occurs when the IV catheter punctures and exits the vein under the skin, causing drugs to infuse or infiltrate into the tissue. Extravasation may happen when the catheter is being inserted or after it is in place if the extremity with the IV catheter is moved or flexed too much. Using a stiff-arm board to prevent excessive movement near the catheter site may help maintain regular flow and prevent extravasation and infiltration. Extravasation and infiltration can be painful and usually requires that the IV be restarted. Some drugs, such as certain chemotherapy agents, may cause severe tissue damage if they infiltrate the tissue. While there are medications to alleviate some of the effects of extravasation and hot and cold compresses to arrest progression, in some cases this tissue damage can be so severe that it requires surgery or even loss of the limb.

- *Particulate matter*—Particulate matter refers to unwanted particles present in parenteral products. Some examples of particulate matter are microscopic glass fragments, hair, lint or cotton fibers, cardboard fragments, undissolved drug particles, and fragments of rubber stoppers, known as cores. Particulate matter that is injected into the bloodstream can cause adverse effects. Improvements in the manufacturing processes have greatly reduced the presence of particulates in commercially available products. Care must be taken in the pharmacy so that particulate matter is not introduced into products. All products should be visually inspected for particulate matter before dispensing. Some institutions may use inline filters to help minimize the amount of particulate that reaches the patient.

- *Pyrogens*—Pyrogens, the by-products or remnants of bacteria, can cause reactions (e.g., fever and chills) if injected in large enough amounts. Because a pyrogen can be present even after a solution has been sterilized, great care must be taken to ensure that these substances are not present.

- *Phlebitis*—Phlebitis, or irritation of the vein, may be caused by the IV catheter, the drug being administered (because of its chemical properties or its concentration), the location of the IV site, a fast rate of administration, or the presence of particulate matter. The patient usually feels pain or discomfort, often severe, along the path of the vein. Red streaking may also occur. If phlebitis is caused by a particular drug, further diluting the drug, then giving it more slowly, or giving it via an IV catheter placed in a vein with a higher, faster-moving volume of blood may be helpful.

Aseptic Preparation of Parenteral Products

As the use of parenteral therapy continues to expand, the need for well-controlled admixture preparation has also grown. Recognizing this need, many pharmacy departments have devoted increased resources to programs that ensure the aseptic preparation of sterile products. The following are the main elements on which these programs focus:[4,5]

- Development and maintenance of good aseptic technique in the personnel who prepare and administer sterile products

- Development and maintenance of a sterile compounding area complete with sterilized equipment and supplies

- Development and maintenance of the skills needed to properly use a laminar airflow hood (LAH)

Aseptic Technique

Aseptic technique is a means of manipulating sterile products without contaminating them. Proper use of an LAH and strict aseptic technique are the most important factors in preventing the contamination of sterile products. Thorough training in the proper use of the LAH and strict aseptic technique, followed by the development of conscientious work habits, is of utmost importance to any sterile products program.

Sterile Compounding Area

Sterile parenteral solutions must be free of living microorganisms and relatively free of particles and pyrogens. Room air typically contains thousands of suspended particles per cubic foot, most of which are too small to be seen with the naked eye. These suspended particles include contaminants such as dust, pollen, smoke, and bacteria. Reducing the number of particles in the air improves the environment in which sterile products are prepared and can be done by following several practices.

A sterile compounding area should be cleaned daily and segregated from normal pharmacy operations, patient specimens, nonessential equipment, and other materials that produce particles. For example, the introduction of cardboard into the clean environment should be avoided. Traffic flow into a clean area should be minimized. Floors should be disinfected periodically, and trash should be removed frequently. Trashcans should be taken outside the IV room before pulling the trash from the container. This will minimize the creation of particulate matter and the risk of spills in the clean room. More sophisticated aspects of clean room design include special filtration or treatment systems for incoming air, ultraviolet irradiation, airlock entry portals, sticky mats to remove particulates from shoes, and positive room air pressure to reduce contaminant entry from adjacent rooms or hallways. Clean rooms are often adjoined by a room, called an *anteroom*, that is used for nonaseptic activities related to the clean room operation, such as order processing, gowning, and stock storage.

Sterile products should be prepared in Class 100 environments, which means environments containing no more than 100 particles per cubic foot that are 0.5 micron or larger in size. LAHs are frequently used to achieve a Class 100 environment.

Laminar Airflow Hoods

The underlying principle of LAHs is that twice-filtered laminar layers of aseptic air continuously sweep the work area inside the hood to prevent the entry of contaminated room air. There are two common types of LAHs: horizontal flow and vertical flow.

Horizontal LAHs—LAHs that sweep filtered air from the back of the hood to the front are called horizontal LAHs (see **Figure 1-4**). Horizontal flow hoods use an electrical blower to draw contaminated room air through a prefilter. The prefilter, which is similar to a furnace filter, removes only gross contaminants and should be cleaned or replaced regularly. The prefiltered air is then pressurized to ensure that a consistent distribution of airflow is presented to the final filtering apparatus. The final filter constitutes the entire back portion of the hood's work area. This *high efficiency particulate air*, or HEPA, filter removes 99.97 percent of particles that are 0.3 micron or larger, thereby elimi-

nating airborne microorganisms, which are usually 0.5 microns or larger.

Vertical LAHs—Laminar flow hoods with a vertical flow of filtered air, are also available. In vertical LAHs, HEPA-filtered air emerges from the top and passes downward through the work area (see Figure 1-4). Because exposure to some antineoplastic (anticancer) drugs may be harmful, these drugs are usually prepared in vertical LAHs to minimize the risk of exposure to airborne drug particulates. The types of vertical LAHs used for the preparation of antineoplastics contain airflow within the hood and are referred to as biological safety cabinets (BSCs).

The critical principle of using LAHs is that nothing must interrupt the flow of air between the HEPA filter and the sterile object. The space between the HEPA filter and the sterile object is known as the *critical area*. The introduction of a foreign object between a sterile

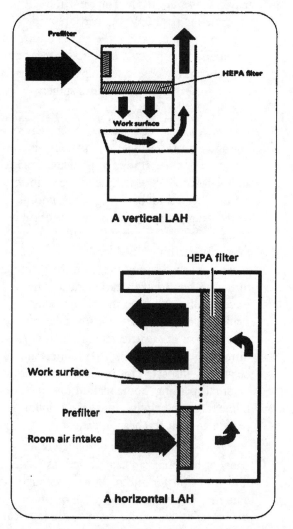

Figure 1-4. Horizontal and vertical laminar airflow hoods with the basic components labeled.

object and the HEPA filter increases wind turbulence in the critical area and the possibility that contaminants from the foreign object may be carried onto the sterile work surface and thereby contaminate an injection port, needle, or syringe. To maintain sterility, nothing should pass behind a sterile object in a horizontal LAH or above a sterile object in a vertical LAH.

Materials placed within the LAH disturb the patterned flow of air blowing from the HEPA filter. The zone of turbulence created behind an object could potentially extend outside the hood, pulling or allowing contaminated room air into the aseptic working area (see **Figure 1-5**). When laminar airflow is moving on all sides of an object, the zone of turbulence extends approximately three times the diameter of that object. When laminar airflow is not accessible to an object on all sides (for example, when placed adjacent to a vertical wall), the zone of turbulence may extend six times the diameter of the object (see **Figure 1-5**). Working with objects at least 6 inches from the sides and front edge of the hood, without blocking air vents is therefore advisable to maintain unobstructed airflow between the HEPA filter and sterile objects. The hands should be positioned so that airflow in the critical area between the HEPA filter and sterile objects is not blocked.

The following are general principles for operating LAHs properly:

- An LAH should be positioned away from excess traffic, doors, air vents, or anything that could produce air currents capable of introducing contaminants into the hood.

- If an LAH is turned off, nonfiltered, nonsterile air will occupy the LAH work area. Therefore,

when it is turned back on, it should be allowed to run for 15 to 30 minutes before it is used (manufacturer recommendations should be consulted for each hood). This time allows the LAH to blow the nonsterile air out of the LAH work area. Then the LAH can be cleaned for use.

- Before using the LAH, all its interior working surfaces should be cleaned with 70 percent isopropyl alcohol or other appropriate disinfecting agent and a clean, lint-free cloth. Cleaning should be performed from the HEPA filter in a side-to-side motion beginning in the rear of the hood and moving toward the front (in a horizontal LAH) so contaminants are moved out of the hood. The hood should be cleaned often throughout the compounding period and when the work surface becomes dirty. Some materials are not soluble in alcohol and may initially require the use of water to be removed. After the water is applied, the surface should be cleaned with alcohol. Plexiglas sides, found on some types of LAHs, should be cleaned with warm, soapy water rather than alcohol. Spray bottles of alcohol should not be used in the LAH, and because they do not allow for the physical action of cleaning the hood, they can damage the HEPA filter, and they do not ensure that alcohol is applied to all areas of the surface to be cleaned. Alcohol should be allowed to dry to increase its effectiveness as a disinfectant.

- Nothing should be permitted to come in contact with the HEPA filter. This includes cleaning solution, aspirate from syringes, or glass from ampules. Ampules should not be opened directly toward the filter.

- Only objects essential to product preparation should be placed in the LAH. Paper, pens, labels, or trays should not be placed in the hood.

- Jewelry should not be worn on the hands or wrists when working in the LAH because it may introduce bacteria or particles into the clean work area.

- Actions such as talking and coughing should be directed away from the LAH working area, and unnecessary motion within the hood should be avoided to minimize the turbulence of airflow.

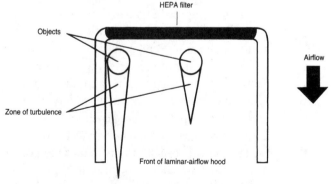

Figure 1-5. Examples of zones of turbulence created behind objects in a horizontal LAH. Notice that the zone of turbulence of the object on the left is greater due to the object's proximity to the side of the hood and has extended outside of the LAH. (Note: figure is not drawn to scale.)

- Smoking, eating, and drinking are prohibited in the aseptic environment.

- All aseptic manipulations should be performed at least 6 inches within the hood to prevent potential contamination caused by the closeness of the worker's body and backwash contamination resulting from turbulent air patterns developing where LAH air meets room air.

- LAHs should be tested by qualified personnel every 6 months, whenever the hood is moved, or if filter damage is suspected. Specific tests are used to certify airflow velocity and HEPA filter integrity.

Although the LAH provides an aseptic environment, safe for the manipulation of sterile products, strict aseptic technique must be used in conjunction with proper hood operation. The use of the LAH alone, without the observance of aseptic technique, cannot ensure product sterility.

Personal Attire

The first component of good aseptic technique is proper personal attire. Clean garments that are relatively particulate free should be worn when preparing sterile products. Clean room attire will depend on institutional policies and is often related to the type of product being prepared. Many facilities provide clean scrub suits or gowns. Scrub suits should not be worn home to ensure that no contaminants are transported home and that the process of cleaning the clothing does not introduce lint onto the low-lint fabric. In addition, suits should be covered up when leaving the pharmacy to minimize the contamination from areas such as the cafeteria. Hair covers, shoe covers, and gloves help reduce particulate or bacterial contamination, and some experts claim that the use of surgical masks is warranted as well. Many facilities also require that all facial hair be covered. The institution's policies regarding facial hair should be consulted.

Handwashing

Touching sterile products while compounding is the most common source of contamination of pharmacy-prepared sterile products. Because the fingers harbor countless bacterial contaminants, proper handwashing is extremely important. The compounder must scrub hands, nails, wrists, and forearms thoroughly for at least 30 seconds with a brush, warm water, and appropriate bactericidal soap before performing aseptic

manipulations and wash hands frequently and every time he or she re-enters the sterile compounding area. Sterile gloves may convey a false sense of security. They are sterile only until they touch something that is not sterile or until they are torn and allow bacteria from the hands to enter the work area. For example, if it is necessary to scratch or touch the face while wearing gloves, the gloves will need to be changed. For these reasons, bare hands should always be washed thoroughly before unwrapping and putting on gloves. Occasionally workers develop allergies to latex as a result of repeated use of latex gloves. Many institutions have now turned to using nonlatex gloves. Workers who have open sores on their hands or have an upper respiratory tract infection should inform their supervisor or consult their institution's quality assurance rules for any special procedures that are warranted.

Equipment and Supplies

Another important factor in aseptic preparation of sterile products is the correct use of appropriate sterile equipment and supplies, including syringes and needles.

Syringes

Syringes are made of either glass or plastic. Most drugs are more stable in glass, so glass syringes are most often used when medication is to be stored in the syringe for an extended period. Some medications may react with the plastics in the syringe, which would alter the potency or stability of the final product. Disposable plastic syringes are most frequently used in preparing sterile products because they are cheaper, durable, and are in contact with substances only for a short time. This minimizes the potential for incompatibility with the plastic itself.

Syringes are composed of a barrel and plunger (see **Figure 1-6**). The plunger, which fits inside the barrel, has a flat disk or lip at one end and a rubber piston at the other. The top collar of the barrel prevents the syringe from slipping during manipulation; the tip is where the needle attaches. To maintain sterility of the product, the syringe tip or the plunger should not be touched. Many syringes have a locking mechanism at the tip, such as the Luer-lock, which secures the needle within a threaded ring. Some syringes, such as slip-tip syringes, do not have a locking mechanism. In this case, friction holds the needle on the syringe.

Syringes are available in numerous sizes, ranging from 0.5 to 60 milliliters (ml). Calibration marks on syringes represent different increments of capacity, depending on the size of the syringe. Usually, the larger the syringe capacity, the larger the interval between calibration lines. For example, each line on a 10 ml syringes represents 0.2 ml, but on a 30 ml syringe, each line represents 1 ml.

To maximize accuracy, the smallest syringe that can hold a desired amount of solution should be used. Syringes are accurate to one-half of the smallest increment marking on the barrel. For example, a 10 ml syringe with 0.2 ml markings is accurate to 0.1 ml and can be used to measure 3.1 ml accurately. A 30 ml syringe with 1 ml markings, however, is only accurate to 0.5 ml and should not be used to measure a volume of 3.1 ml. Ideally, the volume of solution should only take up one-half to two-thirds of the syringe capacity. This avoids inadvertent touch contamination when the syringe plunger is pulled all the way back.

When measuring with a syringe, the final edge (closest to the tip of the syringe) of the plunger piston, which comes in contact with the syringe barrel, should be lined up with the calibration mark on the barrel that corresponds to the volume desired (see **Figure 1-7**).

Syringes are sent from the manufacturer assembled and individually packaged in paper overwraps or plastic covers. The sterility of the contents is guaranteed as long as the outer package remains intact. Therefore, packages should be inspected, and any that are damaged should be discarded. The syringe package should be opened within the LAH to maintain sterility. The wrapper should be peeled apart, not ripped or torn. To minimize particulate contamination, discarded packaging or unopened syringes should not be placed on the LAH work surface.

Syringes may come from the manufacturer with a needle attached or with a protective cover over the syringe tip. The syringe tip protector should be left in place until it is time to attach the needle. For attaching needles to Luer-lock-type syringes, a quarter turn is usually sufficient to secure the needle to the syringe.

Needles

Like syringes, needles are commercially available in many sizes. Sizes are described by two numbers: gauge and length. The gauge of the needle corresponds to the diameter of its bore, which is the diameter of the inside of the shaft. The larger the gauge, the smaller the needle bore. For example, the smallest needles have a gauge of 27, whereas the largest needles have a gauge of 13. The length of a needle shaft is measured in inches and usually ranges from 3/8 to 3 1/2 inches.

The components of a simple needle are the shaft and the hub (see **Figure 1-8**). The hub attaches the needle to the syringe and is often color-coded to correspond to a specific gauge. The tip of the needle shaft is slanted to form a point. The slant is called the *bevel*, and the point is called the *bevel tip*. The opposite end of the slant is called the *bevel heel*.

Needles are sent from the manufacturer individually packaged in paper or plastic overwraps with a protective cover over the needle shaft. This guarantees the sterility as long as the package remains intact. Damaged packages should be discarded.

No part of the needle itself should be touched.

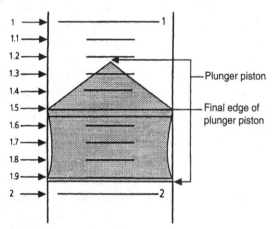

Figure 1-7. A close-up of a syringe showing how to measure 1.5 ml. Note that the final edge of the plunger piston is used to make the measurement.

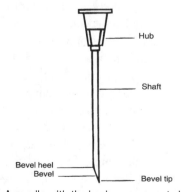

Figure 1-8. A needle with the basic components labeled.

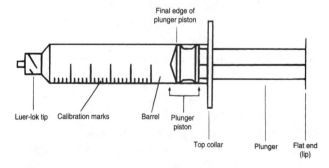

Figure 1-6. A syringe with the basic components labeled.

Needles should be manipulated by their overwrap and protective covers only. The protective cover should be left in place until the needle or syringe is ready to be used. A needle shaft is usually metal and is lubricated with a sterile silicone coating so latex vial tops can be penetrated smoothly and easily. For this reason, needles should never be swabbed with alcohol.

Some needles are designed for special purposes and therefore have unique characteristics. For example, needles designed for batch filling have built-in vents (vented needles) to avoid the need to release pressure that might form in the vial. Another example is needles with built-in filters, meant to be used with products requiring filtering, such as drugs removed from a glass ampule.

Drug Information

Pharmacy technicians are challenged with drug information questions frequently throughout the workday and are called upon to become knowledgeable about the handling, availability, and uses of medications. A basic knowledge of the resources available will make the technician more resourceful and better able to assist the pharmacist with certain drug information requests. Pharmacy reference books and electronic media (including the Internet) that are available in all practice settings often hold answers to typical day-to-day practice-related questions. Before responding to a drug information question, technicians must clearly differentiate questions that fall within their scope of practice from those that must be answered only by a pharmacist. Technicians should identify themselves as pharmacy technicians so the person asking the question will know the type of information that may appropriately be conveyed. If there is any doubt about the nature of the question, the technician should defer the question to the pharmacist. It is important for the technician to learn who the person initiating the request is and to obtain the necessary contact information (phone, fax, pager, etc.) in case the person needs to be called back. The search for, and response to, drug information requests will be different depending on who is requesting the information. Knowing information about the requestor, their training, and their knowledge of the subject will have an impact on what the final response will be and how it will be given. Obtaining background information will help to determine what the needs of the requestor are and will make the search for information more efficient. Background information is especially important to determine if the question pertains to a specific patient or if it is a question that requires interpretation and, therefore, the expertise of a phar-

macist. The urgency of the request and the extent of the information needed should also be determined so an appropriate amount of time is allotted to answer the request. Classifying the type of request helps to narrow the search and makes the search process more efficient. **Table 1-2** lists common types of questions that technicians may get, with examples of each. Technicians should not interpret a patient-specific question or provide information that may require professional judgment. A simply stated question can actually be a complex patient-specific situation. The pharmacist has to find out more about the patient's specific problems and apply clinical judgment to answer the question appropriately. Many times, the person requesting the information may indirectly be asking for a pharmacist's point of view or interpretation of a situation and may thus require an in-depth analysis and recommendation from the pharmacist. Attempting to interpret or answer such a question could result in miscommunication and delivery of inaccurate information. Both scenarios could be potentially harmful to the patient. Examples of questions that require a pharmacist's interpretation and that should not be answered by a technician are provided in **Table 1-3**.

Conducting the Search: Choosing the Right References

The key to answering questions quickly and accurately is knowing where the necessary information is likely to be found. The first step is to consult tertiary references, then secondary references, and finally primary references.

Tertiary references are general references that present documented information in a condensed and compact format. They include textbooks; compendia [e.g., *American Hospital Formulary Service, Drug Information (AHFS DI), Drug Facts and Comparisons*]; computerized systems such as Micromedex® Clinical Information System; review articles; and much of the information found on the Internet. Tertiary references are easy to use, convenient, readily accessible, concise, and compact. Disadvantages of tertiary references are that information may not be timely, the information could contain errors, and may not offer enough information on a specific topic because of space restrictions.

Secondary references include indexing systems such as Medline that provide a list of journal articles on the topic that is being researched. Secondary systems are used when new or very up-to-date information is required or when no information can be found in tertiary references.

TABLE 1-2. TYPES OF DRUG INFORMATION QUESTIONS FOR PHARMACY TECHNICIANS

Classification Type	Examples
General Drug Information	• What is the brand name of warfarin?
	• Do Anaprox® and Aleve® contain the same active ingredient?
	• Who manufactures Enbrel®?
	• Is Claritin® available as a generic? Is it a prescription or over-the-counter (OTC) product?
Availability/Cost	• What dosage forms of Imitrex® are available in your pharmacy?
	• Is Zoloft® available as a liquid? If so, what size and concentration is available?
	• What are the prices of Adalat CC® and Procardia XL®?
	• How long is the shortage of vancomycin oral capsules expected to last?
Storage/Stability	• Should Lovenox® be stored in the refrigerator?
	• How long is a flu shot stable after it is drawn up in a syringe?
Calculations	• How many milliliters are in an ounce?
Preparation	• How should ampicillin be reconstituted?
Pharmacy Law	• In what controlled substance schedule is zolpidem (Ambien®)?
	• Can Tiazac® be substituted for Cardizem CD® (is it AB rated)?
	• How many times can a prescription be transferred from one store to another?
Miscellaneous	• Where can I find the phone number for Aventis?
	• When will the patent for Allegra® expire?
	• Where can I get more Lovenox® teaching kits?

Primary references are original research articles published in scientific journals, such as the *American Journal of Health-System Pharmacy (AJHP)* or the *Journal of the American Pharmacists Association (JAPhA)*.

Other resources include pharmaceutical manufacturers and specialized drug and poison information centers.

If the information cannot be found in a tertiary reference, then the technician should consult a pharmacist, who may advise an alternative search strategy or consult a secondary reference. If time permits, the technician should consult as many resources as possible and compare information among resources.

Common References

Technicians should familiarize themselves with the references in their practice settings to determine which sources best fit their needs. Using a systematic approach when faced with a drug information question will aid in understanding the nature of the request, obtaining pertinent background information, and answering the question. Numerous resources are available to assist with answering drug information requests. Becoming familiar with common resources will make the search process more efficient. It is critical for pharmacy technicians to be able to differentiate between basic drug information questions that they can answer and questions that require clinical judgment and, therefore, should be answered by a pharmacist. The references described in the next few sections are summarized in **Table 1-4** with examples of the types of information one might find in each.

General Drug Information

Drug Facts and Comparisons (published by Facts and Comparisons) is easy to use and available in regularly updated print and electronic versions. It is a comprehensive general drug information reference that provides complete drug monographs. It is organized by therapeutic class (e.g., antihistamines, topicals) and includes tables that allow quick comparisons of drugs within the same class.

United States Pharmacopeia Drug Information [USPDI] *(published by Micromedex)* is a three-volume set that provides medication information for health care professionals (Volume I) and patients (Volume II). The third volume (*Approved Drug Products and Legal Requirements*) provides information on laws affecting pharmacy practice.

TABLE 1-3. TYPES OF DRUG INFORMATION QUESTIONS FOR PHARMACISTS

Classification	Examples	Rationale
Identification and Availability	What is the alternative to Brevital® because of the current shortage?	Although it is appropriate for a technician to get technical information about availability (anticipated length/reasons for a shortage), questions that require clinical knowledge, such as therapeutic alternatives, must be answered by the pharmacist.
Allergies	Which narcotic is safe to use in a patient with a codeine allergy?	For allergy questions, the pharmacist must get more patient-specific information, such as a description of the allergy, what is being treated, etc. Clinical judgment is required.
Dosing and Administration Questions	What is the usual dose of propranolol? How long should ciprofloxacin be given for a urinary tract infection? What is the best way to give gentamicin IV?	Dosing and administration depend on many things, especially the indication for use and patient-specific information (age, weight, kidney and liver function, etc.).
Compatibility	Is Primaxin® compatible with dopamine?	More information is needed (e.g., doses, concentrations, fluids, type of IV lines), and the pharmacist must interpret information found in a reference and apply it to the situation.
Drug Interactions	Is it okay to take aspirin with warfarin?	Drug interaction questions are complex and require patient-specific information and interpretation by the pharmacist to apply the significance of a potential interaction to a specific patient.
Side Effects	What are the side effects of Lexapro®? Can Vioxx® cause renal failure?	Package inserts and textbooks provide lists of side effects that are often difficult to interpret and convey. Also, the pharmacist must interpret whether the question is being asked because an adverse event is suspected with one or more medications.
Pregnancy and Lactation	Is albuterol safe to use in pregnancy? Can I get a flu shot if I am breastfeeding?	Pregnancy and lactation questions are complicated, because more information is needed about the patient as well as the stage of pregnancy or age of the infant. The pharmacist must interpret the findings and apply them to the specific situation.
Therapeutic Use	Has clonidine been used to treat opiate withdrawal?	The use of drugs for off-label uses often requires evaluation and interpretation of the literature and clinical judgment.

TABLE 1-4. REVIEW OF COMMON DRUG INFORMATION REQUESTS AND REFERENCES

Type of Information Needed	Reference Likely to Have Such Information
Product Availability	
• dosage form	American Drug Index
• product strength	Drug Facts and Comparisons
• brand and generic name	Drug Information Handbook
• manufacturer	Internet, PDR
• indication	Micromedex Mosby's Drug Consult
	RedBook (not indication)
	USP DI
Product Identification	
• dosage form	Drug Facts and Comparisons
• product strength	PDR
• brand and generic name	Mosby's Drug Consult
• manufacturer	USP DI
• colored pictures of tablets/capsules	Micromedex
Drug Uses	
• FDA-approved indications	American Hospital Formulary Service
• other uses of the agent	American Drug Index
	Drug Facts and Comparisons
	Drug Information Handbook
	Physicians' Desk Reference (FDA-approved indications only)
	Micromedex
	Mosby's Drug Consult
	USP DI
Drug Monographs	
• general drug information	American Hospital Formulary Service
• pharmacology	Drug Facts and Comparisons
• indications and uses	Drug Information Handbook
• drug interactions	Mosby's Drug Consult
• admixture information	PDR
• doses	USP DI
• adverse effects	Micromedex
• drug interactions	
Injectable Drug Compatibility/Stability Information	
• drug diluent and solution compatibilities	American Hospital Formulary Service
• drug compatibility	Handbook on Injectable Drugs
• conditions for handling products (i.e., glass vs. plastic container, protection from light, filters, refrigeration, expiration, etc.)	Package inserts
	PDR
	Micromedex

cont'd

Type of Information Needed	Reference Likely to Have Such Information
Preparation	*American Hospital Formulary Service*
	Handbook on Injectable Drugs
	Micromedex
	Package inserts
	PDR
Calculations	*American Drug Index*
	Drug Information Handbook
Hazardous Chemicals or Drugs	
• specifies hazards of the chemicals or drugs used at the work site	*Material Safety Data Sheets*
	Micromedex
• guidelines for their safe use	
• recommendations to treat or clean up an exposure	
Pharmacy Law	*USP DI Volume III*
	The Orange Book
Patient Information	*USP DI Volume I*
	Internet (FDA, safemedication.com)
	MedlinePlus
	Micromedex (English and Spanish)
	Patient package inserts

The *Physicians' Desk Reference [PDR] (published by Thomson Medical Economics)* contains manufacturers' package inserts. A package insert is a manufacturer's product information sheet that provides general drug information, such as how the drug works, indications, adverse effects, drug interactions, dosage forms, stability, and dosing information. The *PDR* is not comprehensive and contains information only on select brand name drugs. The information is written by the manufacturer and approved by the FDA. It contains only information about FDA-approved uses of the drug and does not provide information comparing that drug with similar medications. Therefore, using the *PDR* to compare products is not as straightforward as using other reference books.

American Hospital Formulary Service Drug Information [AHFS DI] (published by the American Society of Health-System Pharmacists, ASHP) is a detailed, comprehensive, general drug information reference. This textbook provides complete drug monographs that are organized by therapeutic class (e.g., anti-infectives, cardiovascular). It provides detailed information about the use of a drug, its side effects, dosing considerations, and so on, and its coverage is not limited to FDA-approved uses of medications. It is especially useful for preparation and administration instructions for injectable products.

Lexi-Comp's Drug Information Handbook and *Drug Information Handbook for the Allied Health Professional (published by Lexi-Comp)* are handbooks containing general drug information monographs. They are widely used because they are quick, convenient, and easy to use. The *Drug Information Handbook* is alphabetically organized in dictionary format according to generic name. The *Drug Information Handbook for the Allied Health Professional* is not as comprehensive as the *Drug Information Handbook*, but it may be appealing to technicians because it allows quick access to basic data on the most frequently used medications. Both publications contain extensive appendixes with helpful charts, abbreviations, measurements, and conversions.

Mosby's Drug Consult (published by Elsevier Science) is a comprehensive general drug information reference. It provides complete drug monographs that are organized alphabetically by generic drug names. This textbook is more comprehensive than the *PDR*. A key feature is its indexing system, which allows identification of all drugs within a therapeutic class, schedules of controlled substances, pregnancy categories, and so on.

American Drug Index (published by Facts and Comparisons) is an alphabetical listing of drugs with brief information on each agent, including drug name (generic, brand, chemical name), manufacturer, dosage form, strength and packaging information, and general uses (e.g., general anesthetic, narcotic, antitussive). It also contains pharmaceutical manufacturers' phone numbers and addresses, weight and measuring conversions, and a list of drugs that should not be crushed. Its extensive cross-indexing is useful to quickly identify a brand or generic product or determine product availability information.

Micromedex® Healthcare Series is a comprehensive reference system that is accessed electronically via CD-ROM, Internet, or personal digital assistant (PDA). Depending on the subscription, it contains comprehensive drug information, poison information, foreign drug information, tablet and capsule identification, disease and trauma information, herbal information, stability information, compatibility information, pregnancy information, patient information, and more. Unfortunately, the cost of the subscription prohibits many pharmacy settings from purchasing this system.

Availability/Cost

Red Book (published by Medical Economics) contains up-to-date product information and prices for prescription drugs, over-the-counter products, and medical supplies. It contains National Drug Code (NDC) numbers for all products, available packaging, and therapeutic equivalence ratings (according to the FDA's *Orange Book*). It has a comprehensive listing of manufacturers, wholesalers, and third-party administrator directories. There are sections with other useful practical information, such as lists of sugar-, lactose-, galactose-, and alcohol-free products; sulfite-containing products; medications that should not be crushed; and color photographs of many prescription and over-the-counter products.

Compatibility and Stability

Trissel's Handbook on Injectable Drugs (published by American Society of Health-System Pharmacists, ASHP) is a textbook often used in hospital and home health care pharmacies. It focuses solely on injectable medications. Information includes data on the solubility, compatibility, and stability of many different medications. Specifically, this handbook is useful to determine when two medications may be safely mixed together in an IV bag, a syringe, or at a Y-site on an administration set. This reference also addresses special handling requirements of certain agents (glass vs. plastic containers, light restrictions, filters, refrigeration requirements, expiration, etc.).

Miscellaneous References

Material Safety Data Sheets are information sheets provided by manufacturers for chemicals or drugs that may be hazardous in the workplace. The primary purpose of the MSDS is to provide information about the specific hazards of the chemicals or drugs (i.e., to describe acute and chronic health effects), guidelines for their safe use, and recommendations to treat an exposure or clean up a spill.

The Internet

The technician must take care to ensure that the information is current and up-to-date and that it is accurate and from a reputable source. Generally, Web sites that are sponsored by the government, pharmacy and medical organizations, and medical centers are the most reputable. **Table** 1-5 lists useful Web sites for drug

information and a brief description of what each site contains.

Billing Methods

Third-party Payment Programs for Ambulatory Pharmacy

One of the most time-consuming activities in the ambulatory care pharmacy setting is dealing with third-party payment programs. Third-party programs are insurance or entitlement programs that reimburse the pharmacy for products delivered and services rendered. Although hundreds of third-party programs are administered by organizations ranging from large insurance companies to small employer or union-sponsored employee benefit programs, there are only two major mechanisms for pharmacy reimbursement: fee-for-service and capitation.

Fee-for-service
In a fee-for-service system, patients pay cash for the

TABLE 1-5. USEFUL WEB SITES FOR OBTAINING DRUG INFORMATION		
Web Site	**Address**	**Description**
Food and Drug Administration	www.fda.gov	Home page for the FDA; contains numerous useful links for both consumers and health care professionals.
FDA Center for Drug Evaluation and Research (CDER)	www.fda.gov/cder	Contains links for consumer and health care professionals regarding drug information, such as new drug approvals, drug shortages, safety information, and generic drug bioequivalence.
Centers for Disease Control and Prevention (CDC)	www.cdc.gov	Home page for the CDC; contains information about diseases, health topics, vaccines, traveler's health, bioterrorism, etc.
National Institutes of Health (NIH)	www.nih.gov	Home page for the NIH; contains information about health topics, clinical trials, and the various divisions of the NIH.
FDA Consumer Information	www.fda.gov/cder/consumerinfo	Contains FDA-approved patient drug information from January 1998 to the present. Also contains a link to the manufacturers' package inserts.
National Library of Medicine/ Medline/PubMed and MedlinePlus	www.nlm.nih.gov	Home page for the U.S. National Library of Medicine. Links to Medline Plus (health information for consumers) and Medline/ PubMed (references and abstracts from biomedical journals).
American Society for Health-System Pharmacists (ASHP)	www.ashp.org	Home page for ASHP; contains news related to health-system pharmacy and many helpful links for pharmacy professionals.
ASHP Drug Shortages Resource Center	www.ashp.org/shortage	Up-to-date information on current drug shortages, including which products are affected and why, the anticipated time to resolution, and alternatives.
ASHP Consumer Drug Information	www.safemedication.com	Reputable site for patient medication information.
American Pharmaceutical Association (APhA)	www.aphanet.org	Home page for APhA; contains news related to pharmacy and many helpful links for pharmacy professionals.
Virtual Library Pharmacy	www.pharmacy.org	Contains links to pharmacy associations, pharmaceutical manufacturers, government sites, hospitals, journals and books, and more.

prescription and submit receipts to their insurance carrier. Alternatively, the pharmacy bills the insurance carrier directly each time eligible products are dispensed or services rendered; the insurance carrier then reimburses the pharmacy. The amount charged and amount reimbursed depends on the cost and time involved. For patients without insurance, this is an "out-of-pocket" expense.

Capitation

Under a capitated payment program, the pharmacy receives a set amount of money for a defined group of patients, regardless of the number of prescriptions or amount of services rendered. The dollar amount is usually in terms of per patient per month. For example, the third-party payer may agree to pay the pharmacy $2 per member per month. Therefore, if the program has 100 patients, the pharmacy receives $200 each month. Even if one of the patients does not use the pharmacy, the pharmacy still receives $2 for that patient. Likewise, if a patient receives multiple medications and uses the pharmacy 10 times per month, the pharmacy still receives only $2 for that patient. The concept of capitation was popular in the 1990s but rarely implemented. Today, very little capitation exists at the pharmacy level.

Copayments/Deductibles/Spend-downs

Third parties designate three basic copayment arrangements: flat rate, variable rate, and straight percentage. A flat rate requires a specific copay regardless of the cost of the drug. A variable-rate copay changes depending on the cost of the drug. In perhaps its simplest form, the variable-rate copay is higher for brand name products and less for generics. Today, a popular version of the variable-rate copay is the multitier copay. The copay in this instance may be low for a generic, mid-level for a brand product on formulary, and high for a brand name off formulary. For instance, the copay structure may be $5.00, $10.00, and $25.00, respectively.

A straight percentage copay requires the patient to pay a percentage of the total cost of the medication. The amount the patient pays increases as the cost of the prescriptions increases. For instance, if the copay is 10 percent, the patient pays $10.00 for a $100.00 prescription or $20 for a $200.00 prescription.

A spend-down (also known as a front-end deductible) differs from a copay or deductible in that it is assessed over a defined period of time and not on a per prescription basis. A spend-down requires a patient to spend a defined amount of out-of-pocket dollars on prescriptions within a year before the third party pays anything. For example, a patient may have a spend-down of $500 over 1 year. This patient will have to buy $500 worth of prescription drugs (out-of-pocket) first, and then the third party will pay for the remaining prescriptions during the rest of the year.

Most prescription plans allow for "on-line adjudication" of prescriptions. This process verifies the patient's eligibility, identifies the reimbursement type, and identifies any fee due from the patient at the time of purchase.

Billing Methods in Institutional Pharmacy

Most billing in institutional settings is imbedded within the patient's overall bill for the stay. The patient's bill must, however, accurately reflect the medications that were administered. Most institutional pharmacies have some type of computerized billing system that automatically transfers a charge for medications to the patient's bill. Which system performs this function and at what point in the process the transfer happens may vary. There are three basic systems: billing at the time of order entry, billing at the time of dispensing, and billing at the time of administration.

Billing at the time of order entry charges the dispensed quantity of medication to the patient as soon as the order is entered by the pharmacy. Subsequent charges are transmitted every time the order is refilled for the patient. Some order entry charges assume a "flat rate charge" for the use or availability of the medication. A flat rate might occur, for example, on an order for a sliding scale insulin, rather than a charge for each administration. The flat rate is generally based on average usage for the order type.

Billing at the time of dispensing is a common method in many institutions that use point-of-care dispensing technology, such as Omnicell® or Pyxis®. The medication, rather than being charged at the time of order entry, is charged when withdrawn from the machine. This system may make billing more accurate by eliminating charges for lost medications. It also eliminates a lot of the crediting activity created when medications are returned to the pharmacy unused after being billed at the time of order entry.

Billing at the time of administration is the most accurate and efficient of the three. This system can be used when bedside bar-code recognition of the patient and the medication allows for billing to be transmitted by the bar-code reader. It virtually eliminates crediting processes in the pharmacy and charges patients only for medications they actually receive.

Transferring Prescriptions

The laws regarding the transfer of prescriptions between pharmacies vary among states and among different classes of drugs. However, the pharmacist is always ultimately responsible for the information transferred. The transfer of a prescription to another pharmacy is usually initiated by a phone call from the pharmacy needing a transferred prescription. A technician may pull the original prescription from files or pull up the data on the computer, but the actual transfer of information is usually the responsibility of the pharmacist.

The same is true for prescriptions being transferred into the pharmacy. In this case, the process begins when a patient requests to transfer the prescription from another location. At that point, the technician must obtain from the patient as much information as possible about the prescription. At a minimum, the pharmacist needs the patient's name and the name of the pharmacy currently holding the prescription. If a patient brings in an old container, it may be useful to troubleshoot the label. For example, if the label indicates that there are no refills, the physician will have to be called to authorize the refill.

References

1. The United States Pharmacopeia, 27th rev. ed., and the national formulary, 22nd ed. Rockville, MD: The United States Pharmacopeial Convention Inc; 2004:2346.

2. The United States Pharmacopeia, 27th rev. ed., and the national formulary, 22nd ed. Rockville, MD: The United States Pharmacopeial Convention Inc; 2004:2349.

3. Anon. ASHP gears up multistep action plan regarding sterile drug products. *Am J Hosp Pharm*. 1991; 48:386, 389–90. News.

4. Dugleaux G, Coutour XL, Hecquard C, et al. Septicemia caused by contaminated parenteral nutrition pouches: the refrigerator as an unusual cause. *JPEN*. 1991; 15:474–5.

5. Solomon SL, Khabbaz RF, Parker RH, et al. An outbreak of Candida parapsilosis bloodstream infections in patients receiving parenteral nutrition. *J Infect Dis*. 1984; 149:98–102.

Suggested Reading

From *Manual for Pharmacy Technicians*, 3rd ed.

Medical Terminology and Abbreviations: See Chapter 8—Medical Terminology and Abbreviations.

Processing Medication Orders and Prescriptions: See Chapter 9—Interpreting Medication Orders and Prescriptions.

Compounding: See Chapter 13—Nonsterile Compounding and Repackaging, Chapter 14—Aseptic Technique, Sterile Compounding, and Intravenous Admixture Programs, and Chapter 4—Home Care Pharmacy Practice.

Drug Information: See Chapter 17—Introduction to Drug Information Resources.

Ambulatory Billing Methods: See Chapter 9—Interpreting Medication Orders and Prescriptions, and Chapter 2—Ambulatory Care Pharmacy.

Transferring Prescriptions: See Chapter 6—Pharmacy Law.

Self-Assessment Questions

1. Abbreviations are generally considered to be unsafe and should therefore never be used in prescriptions.
   a. True
   b. False

2. The first step in receiving either a prescription or a medication order is to verify that all necessary information is present, although this information may vary depending on the pharmacy site (outpatient versus inpatient).
   a. True
   b. False

3. The abbreviation for "at bedtime" is
   a. b.t.
   b. qid
   c. hs
   d. ac
   e. rx

4. Which piece of information is critical in an ambulatory pharmacy environment when filling a prescription but is often not known by the pharmacy in a hospital?
   a. patient's allergies
   b. name of the ordered drug
   c. dose of the ordered drug
   d. patient's insurance information
   e. name of the doctor

5. Which reference is important in describing good compounding practices for technicians?
   a. Lexi-Comp's *Drug Information Handbook for the Allied Health Professional*
   b. Micromedex
   c. Package inserts
   d. *PDR*
   e. *USP 27*

6. Which of the following is a possible risk associated with IV therapy?
   a. infection
   b. bleeding
   c. air embolus
   d. incompatibilities
   e. all of the above

7. Which of the following is false regarding the use of a Laminar Airflow Hood (LAH)?
   a. Hoods should be allowed to run for 15–30 minutes before use if they are not left on continuously.

   b. All compounding should be done at least 3 inches from the front edge of the hood.
   c. Only essential objects should be taken into the hood.
   d. Jewelry should not be worn on the hands or wrists when working in the hood.
   e. Actions such as talking or coughing should be directed from the LAH work area.

8. Which question can a pharmacy technician answer?
   a. When will the shortage of methylprednisolone be over?
   b. How much ibuprofen should I give my 2 month old infant?
   c. Can acetaminophen make me dizzy?
   d. Does verapamil interact with grapefruit juice?
   e. What should I substitute for morphine if my patient is allergic?

9. Which reference has the best information about IV compatibility?
   a. *American Drug Index*
   b. *PDR*
   c. *Drug Facts and Comparisons*
   d. Package inserts
   e. *Handbook on Injectable Drugs*

10. Every state's laws regarding prescription transfer are the same.
    a. True
    b. False

Self-Assessment Answers

1. b
2. a
3. c
4. d
5. e
6. e
7. b
8. a
9. e
10. b

Medication Distribution and Inventory Control Systems

2

The Formulary System

Most hospitals and health care systems develop a list of medications that may be prescribed for their patients. This list, usually called a *formulary*, serves as the cornerstone of the purchasing and inventory control system. The formulary is developed and maintained by a committee of medical and allied health staff called the Pharmacy and Therapeutics (P&T) Committee. This group generally consists of physicians, pharmacists, nurses, and administrators, although other disciplines may be present, including dieticians, risk managers, and case managers. The group collaborates to ensure that the safest, most efficacious, and least costly medications are included on the formulary. The products on the hospital formulary dictate what the hospital pharmacy should keep in inventory. Third-party prescription drug benefit providers will also establish plan-specific formularies for their ambulatory patients. Ambulatory (retail) pharmacy staff frequently encounter insurance plan–specific drug formularies in serving their customers and adjust their inventory accordingly. Most retail pharmacies do not restrict items in their inventory rigidly. This is because in this setting, inventories are largely dependent on the dynamic needs of their patient population and, to some degree, the patients' insurance plans. Therefore, the concept of formulary management differs greatly depending on the perspective (i.e., that of the hospital compared with that of the retail pharmacy).

Ordering Pharmaceuticals

Some pharmacies employ a dedicated purchasing agent to manage the procurement and inventory of pharmaceuticals. Others employ a more general approach whereby a variety of staff are involved in ordering pharmaceuticals. The state-of-the-art practice involves the use of computer and Internet technology to manage the process of purchasing and receiving pharmaceuticals from a drug wholesaler. This process includes online procurement and purchase order generation and electronic receiving processes that involve bar-code technology and hand-held computer devices. Use of computer technology for these purposes has many benefits, including up-to-the-minute product availability information, comprehensive reporting capabilities, accuracy, and efficiency. Use of computer technology also facilitates compliance with various pharmaceutical purchasing contracts.

Learning Objectives

After completing this chapter, the technician should be able to

1. Describe distribution processes used in the inpatient and outpatient setting.

2. Explain the role of the formulary in purchasing and inventory systems.

3. Describe the methods of inventory control that may be used to maintain adequate stocks of pharmaceuticals and medical devices.

4. Explain the ordering, receiving, and stocking process for pharmaceuticals and medical devices.

5. Describe inventory procedures for recalled products, controlled substances, investigational drugs, and other products requiring special handling.

Receiving and Storing Pharmaceuticals

One of the most useful experiences for a new pharmacy technician is to witness the receipt of pharmaceuticals by the pharmacy department. This experience is useful for a number of reasons: It helps the pharmacy technician become familiar with various processes involved with the ordering and receipt of pharmaceuticals; it may help the technician become familiar with formulary items; it may demonstrate the system used to ensure that only formulary items are put into inventory; and it helps familiarize the technician with the locations in which drugs are stored.

Receiving is one of the most important parts of the pharmacy operation. A poorly organized and executed receiving system can put patients at risk and elevate health care costs. For example, if the wrong concentration of a product were received in error, it could lead to a dosing error or a delay in therapy. Misplaced products or out-of-stock products jeopardize patient care as well as the efficiency of the pharmacy —both undesirable and costly outcomes. To avoid these unfavorable outcomes, pharmacy technicians should become familiar with the process for receiving and storing pharmaceuticals.

The Receiving Process

Some pharmacies create processes whereby, as much as is possible, the person receiving pharmaceuticals is different from the individual ordering them. This is especially important for controlled substances because it effectively establishes a check in the system to minimize opportunities for drug diversion.

In a reliable and efficient receiving system, the receiving personnel verify that the shipment is complete and intact (i.e., check for missing or damaged items) before putting items into circulation or inventory. The receiving process begins with the verification of the boxes containing pharmaceuticals delivered by the shipper. The person receiving the shipment verifies that the name and address on the boxes is correct and that the number of boxes matches the shipping manifest. Many drug wholesalers use rigid plastic crates because they protect the contents of each shipment better than foam or cardboard boxes. Plastic crates are also environmentally friendly because they are returned to the wholesaler for cleaning and reuse. In any case, each box should be inspected for gross damage.

Products with a cold storage requirement (i.e., refrigeration or freezing) should be processed first (see **Table 2-1** for storage temperatures). The shipper is responsible for ensuring the cold storage environment is maintained during shipping and will generally package these items in a transportable foam cooler. The shipper will include frozen cold packs to keep products at the correct storage temperature during shipment.

Receiving personnel play a critical role in protecting the pharmacy from financial responsibility for products damaged in shipment, products not ordered, and products not received. If there is any obvious damage or other discrepancies with the shipment, such as a breech in the cold storage environment or an incorrect product, they should be noted on the shipping manifest and, if warranted, the appropriate part of the shipment should be refused. Ideally, gross shipment damage or incorrect box counts should be identified in the presence of the delivery person and should be documented when signing for the order. Other problems identified after delivery personnel have left, such as mispicks, product dating, or internally damaged goods, must be resolved according to the vendor's policies. Most vendors have specific procedures to follow in reporting and resolving such problems.

TABLE 2-1. DEFINED STORAGE TEMPERATURES AND HUMIDITY†		
Freezer	-25° to -10° C	-13° to 14° F
Cold (Refrigerated)	2° to 8° C	36° to 46° F
Cool	8° to 15° C	46° to 59° F
Room Temperature	The temperature prevailing in a working area.	
Controlled Room Temperature	20° to 25 C	68° to 77° F
Warm	30° to 40° C	86° to 104° F
Excessive Heat	Any temperature above 40° C (104° F)	
Dry Place	A place that does not exceed 40% average relative humidity at controlled room temperature or the equivalent water vapor pressure at other temperatures. Storage in a container validated to protect the article from moisture vapor, including storage in bulk, is considered a dry place.	

† United States Pharmacopeia 26/The National Formulary 21. Rockville, MD: United States Pharmacopeial Convention, Inc.; 2003:9–10.

PURCHASE ORDER
Department of Pharmacy Services
Community Hospital
1 Valley Road
Suburbia, MD 20777
(333) 555-1010

Purchase Order
No. 0849
THIS NUMBER MUST
APPEAR ON ALL INVOICES,
PACKING SLIPS, BILLS,
PACKAGES AND CARTONS

Vendor: Pharmaceutical Labs
           185 Commerce Ave.
           Ft. Washington, PA
           1-800-555-3753
           Acc# 123-12345

BY_____DIRECTOR
PHARMACY SERVICES/DESIGNEE

ORDER DATE 4/1/97	FOB ☐ HOSPITAL ☐ SHIPPING POINT	DATE REQUIRED IN HOSPITAL ASAP	TERMS N/A	DEPARTMENT Pharmacy	SHIP VIA Standard

QUANTITY RECEIVED	ORDERED	DESCRIPTION	UNIT PRICE	AMOUNT
4	5	Orimune 50 × 1	$450.00	$2,250.00
50	50	Haemophilus B Vaccine Via 4s	$ 52.92	
13	12	Piperacillin 40 g Vial each	$110.00	$2,646.00
30	30	DPT Vaccine Vial 7.5 ml each	$ 56.50	
		Quantity received as indicated / one vial of Piperacillin broken in shipment.		$1,320.00
				$1,695.00
		4/15/97 Joe Johnson, Pharmacy Technician		

1. Goods not in accordance with specifications will be rejected and held at vendor's risk awaiting disposal. Vendor must pay transportation both ways on all rejected material.
2. The right is reserved to cancel all or part of this order if not delivered within the time specified.
3. No price change allowed unless authorized by this office.
4. Packing slips must accompany all shipments.
5. All shipments must be prepaid.
6. Equipment supplied under this purchase order must meet all applicable O.S.H.A.. Standards.

The quantity received is recorded in the "received" column by the person receiving the order. Damaged merchandise is noted on the purchase order, and the receiver signs and dates the receipt. This information enables the purchasing agent to confirm back orders, address mechanisms for retaining or returning overages, and determine financial accountability for damaged merchandise.

Figure 2-1. Documenting Receipt on a Purchase Order

The next step of the receiving process entails checking the newly delivered products against the receiving copy of the purchase order. This generally occurs after the delivery person has left. A *purchase order*, created when the order is placed, is a complete list of the items that were ordered. Traditionally, a purchase order is executed in multiple copies, including an original file copy, a copy used in the receiving process, and a copy for the supplier (see **Figure 2-1** previous page).

The person responsible for checking products into inventory uses the receiving copy to ensure that the products ordered have been received. The name, brand, dosage form, size of the package, concentration strength, and quantity of product must match the purchase order. Generally, once the accuracy of the shipment is confirmed, the purchase order copy is signed and dated by the person receiving the shipment (Figure 2-1). At this point, the product's expiration date should be checked to ensure that it meets the pharmacy's minimum expiration date requirement. Frequently, pharmacies will require that products received have a minimum 6 months' shelf life remaining before they expire. It is worth mentioning that, on occasion, the manufacturer or wholesaler may unintentionally ship an excess quantity of a product to the pharmacy. The ethical response is to notify the manufacturer or wholesaler of this situation immediately and arrange for the return of any excess quantity.

Controlled substances require additional processing upon receipt. Regulations specific to Schedule II controlled substances require the completion of DEA form 222 upon receipt of these products. The form must be filed separately with a copy of the invoice and packing slip accompanying each shipment. If a pharmacist or pharmacy technician other than the receiving technician removes a product from a shipment before it has been properly received and cannot locate the receiving copy of the purchase order, then a written record of receipt should be created. This is done by listing the product, dosage form, concentration or strength, package size, and quantity on a blank piece of paper (see **Figure 2-2**) or on the supplier's packing slip

or invoice and checking off the line item received (see **Figure 2-3**). In both cases, the name of the person receiving the product should be included and the document should be given to the receiving technician to avoid confusion and an unnecessary call to the wholesaler or manufacturer.

The Storing Process

Once the product has been properly received, it must be properly stored. Depending on the size and type of the pharmacy operation, the product may be placed in a bulk central storage area or in the active dispensing areas of the pharmacy. In any case, the expiration date of the product should be compared with the products currently in stock. Products in stock that have expired should be removed. Products that will expire in the near future should be highlighted and placed in the front of the shelf or bin. This is a common practice known as *stock rotation*. The newly acquired products will generally have longer shelf lives and should be placed behind products that will expire before them. Stock rotation is an important inventory management principle that promotes the use of products before they expire and helps prevent the use of expired products and waste.

Product Handling Considerations

Pharmacy technicians usually spend more time handling and preparing medications than do pharmacists.

Invoice

Shipper	Buyer
Pharmaceutical Labs	Community Hospital
185 Commerce Avenue	1 Valley Road
Ft. Washington, PA	Suburbia, MD 20777

Invoice # 12346
Invoice Date 4/01/97

Quantity		Product #	Product Description	Unit Price	Amount
5	4 rec.	6190	Orimune 50 × 1	$450.00	$2,250.00
4	✓	7183	Haemophilus B Vaccine	$ 52.92	$2,646.00
13	12. rec.	4391	Piperacillin 40 g Vial	$110.00	$1,320.00
30	✓	2727	DPT Vaccine 7.5ml Vial	$ 56.50	$1,695.00

Quantity received as indicated.
one vial Piperacillin broken in shipment.

Received 4 × 50's Orimune
50   Haemophilus B Vaccine.
13   Piperacillin 40 gm vial
30   DTP Vaccine 7.5 ml
4/15/97
Joe Johnson
Pharmacy Technician

Figure 2-3. Receipt of Pharmaceutical on Packing Slip/Invoice

Received to stock
4 × 50's Oral Polio Vaccine, 0.5 ml
50 × 4's Haemophilus B vaccine vials
13 each Piperacillin 40 gm vials
30   DTP vials, 7.5 ml
4/15/97
Joe Johnson
Pharmacy Technician
One vial Piperacillin broken in shipment.

Figure 2-2. Receipt of Pharmaceutical on Blank Piece of Paper

This situation presents pharmacy technicians with the critical responsibility of assessing and evaluating each product from both a content and labeling standpoint. It also gives technicians an opportunity to confirm that the receiving process was performed properly.

Just as checking the product label carefully at the time a prescription or medication order is filled is important, so is taking the same care when receiving and storing pharmaceuticals. It is best to read product packaging carefully rather than rely on the general appearance of the product (e.g., packaging type, size or shape, color, logo), because a product's appearance may change frequently and may be similar to other products. Technicians play a vital role in minimizing dispensing errors caused by human fallibility. Technicians are generally the first in a series of double checks involved in an accurate dispensing process.

When performing purchasing or inventory management roles, the technician must pay close attention to the product's expiration date. For liquids or injectable products, color and clarity should also be checked for consistency with the product standard. Products with visible particles, an unusual appearance, or a broken seal should be reported to the pharmacist.

Because pharmacy technicians handle so many products each day, they are in a perfect position to identify packaging and storage issues that could lead to errors. Technicians must pay close attention to three main issues:

- *Look-Alike/Sound-Alike Products.* Stocking products of similar color, shape, and size could result in error if someone fails to read the label carefully. All staff members should be alerted to look-alike or sound-alike products.
- *Misleading Labels.* Sometimes the company name or logo is emphasized on the label instead of the drug name, concentration, or strength.
- *Product Storage.* Storing products that are similar in appearance next to one another can result in error if someone fails to read the label.

Alerting other staff members to products that fall into one of these categories is essential. Some pharmacies routinely discuss product-handling considerations at staff meetings or in departmental newsletters. Dispensing errors may be averted by simply relocating a look-alike/sound-alike product to a different shelf location or placing warning notes (i.e., auxiliary labeling or highlights) on the shelf or on the product itself. Pharmacy technicians should also discuss their concerns with coworkers and may advocate changes to products with poor labeling with the manufacturer.

Maintaining and Managing Inventory

An inventory management system is an organized approach designed to maintain just the right amount of pharmaceutical products in the pharmacy at all times. A variety of inventory management systems are in use, ranging from simple to complex. They include the order book, the minimum/maximum (par) level, the Pareto (ABC) analysis, economic order quantity (EOQ), and, finally, the fully automated, computerized system.

Economic Models

The Pareto ABC system, also known as the *80/20 rule,* relies on the premise that managing 20 percent of the inventory will cover 80 percent of the costs. It essentially groups inventory products by aggregate value and volume of use into three groupings (A, B, and C). This analysis is useful to determine where inventory control efforts are best directed. For example, Group A may include 10 percent of all items that make up 70 percent of the inventory cost. Tight control over these items would be sensible. Group B may include 20 percent of items that make up 15 percent of the inventory cost. An automatic order cycle here based on well-established par levels (see below) might be useful. Group C may include 70 percent of items that make up 10 percent of the inventory cost. Less aggressive monitoring of these items may be justifiable.

The EOQ, also known as the *Minimum Cost Quantity* approach, is a model for calculating inventory order quantities. In essence, EOQ is an accounting formula used to determine the point at which the combination of order costs and inventory holding costs are minimized. One variation of the EOQ formula is as follows:

$$EOQ = \sqrt{\frac{2(\text{Annual usage in units})(\text{Order cost})}{(\text{Annual carrying cost per unit})}}$$

The EOQ relies heavily on the accuracy of various data inputs, such as annual product usage, fixed costs associated with each order (including processing the purchase order, receiving, inspection, processing the invoice, vendor payment, and inbound freight costs), and the annual cost per average on-hand inventory unit. If calculated accurately, it results in the most cost-efficient order quantity. Economists would argue that anytime one has repetitive purchasing tasks, EOQ should be considered. It is relatively difficult to apply this model universally in pharmacy practice due to the wide variability of the individual patient's pharmaceutical needs. Therefore, some pharmacies may choose to use a combination of the systems mentioned here.

Automation

The ideal system for inventory management is an automated or computerized system that supports a *just-in-time* product inventory. Just-in-time inventory management is a philosophy that simply means products are ordered and delivered at just the right time—when they are needed for patient care, with a goal of minimizing wasted steps, labor, and cost. Pharmaceuticals are neither overstocked nor understocked. In pharmacy, this business philosophy couples responsible financial management of pharmaceutical purchasing with the clinical aspects of patient care. A related business philosophy is known as *maximizing inventory turns*. The philosophy is that a product should not sit on the shelf, unused, for long periods of time. Ideally, specific drug inventory is purchased and used many times throughout the course of a year. A simple means of calculating inventory turns in a given period is to divide the total purchases in that period by the value of physical inventory taken at one point in time. For example, if total pharmaceutical purchases for fiscal year 2004 were $10,243,590 and the physical inventory value on 12/31/2003 was $521,550, the calculated inventory turns for fiscal year 2004 would be 19.6 times ($10,243,590/$521,550 = 19.6). This method assumes a relatively constant volume of pharmaceutical purchases and constant residual inventory over time. The economic principle is simple: One does not want to buy pharmaceuticals that won't be used in a timely manner. Minimizing inventory carrying costs (or holding costs) is an important aspect of sound business administration. *Carrying cost* can be defined as all costs associated with inventory investment and storage costs. It might include interest, insurance, taxes, and storage expenses.

Although automated inventory management modalities are available, they are not the mainstay in practice today. Many pharmacies still use a manual inventory management system. Manual systems require the active oversight of pharmacy technicians and are usually based on a minimum/maximum, or par-level, system. Staff may create a pharmaceutical order through the use of a handheld bar-code scanning device or may enter product stock numbers directly into a PC. Manual systems typically involve a minimum/maximum, or par-level, shelf-sticker that corresponds to each product. The minimum and maximum inventory level is written on this label and the information is used as a relative guide for pharmacy staff

involved in purchasing. Staff strive to maintain pharmaceutical inventories within the minimum and maximum range to avoid both overstocking and understocking. Overstocking exposes the pharmacy to unnecessary expense, and understocking may affect patient care.

This minimum/maximum system requires pharmacy staff to routinely scan inventory levels and place orders accordingly. With either electronic or manual systems, pharmacy staff should realize that the diversity of their patients' needs may require modification in a particular product's par level. In the fully computerized inventory system, each dispensing transaction is subtracted from the perpetual inventory log that is maintained electronically in the computer, and all products received are added to the inventory log. When the quantity of a pharmaceutical product in stock reaches a predetermined point (often called *par* or *par level*), a purchase order is automatically generated to order more of the product. The system does not depend on any one employee to monitor the inventory or to reorder pharmaceuticals. The technology is available to have a computerized inventory in most pharmacies, yet a computerized inventory system that interfaces with existing pharmacy computer systems designed for dispensing and patient management systems is often difficult to implement. Additionally, other variables, such as product availability, contract changes, and changing use patterns (either up or down), make relying on the fully computerized model challenging. Consequently, even the most sophisticated electronic or automated systems require human oversight.

The minimum/maximum (par) level inventory system relies on a predetermined order quantity and an order point. Shelf labels are placed on the storage bin or shelf to alert all staff to the minimum stock quantity (see **Figure 2-4**). The pharmacy technician should always determine if the minimum stock quantity has been reached when removing a product and should then

Figure 2-4. Shelf Labels

inform the appropriate purchasing personnel or list the item on a designated order book as described below. An assigned staff member performs a periodic inventory of the stock to identify those products that have a stock level at or below the reorder point. When the inventory is reduced to or below the order point, designated pharmacy personnel initiate a purchase order or electronically transmit a purchase order to a drug wholesaler.

Many pharmacies use an order book system, also called a *want list* or *want book*. When pharmacists or pharmacy technicians determine that a product should be reordered, they write the item in the order book. Although this approach is simple, it also provides the least amount of organized control over inventory. Its success is highly dependent on the participation of staff. Therefore, it is usually not the sole method of inventory management and is often used in conjunction with one of the other systems mentioned.

The use of automated dispensing devices in inpatient hospital nursing units, clinics, operating rooms, and emergency rooms has facilitated the use of computers for inventory management. Similar devices are evolving for the retail pharmacy and hold promise for making the dispensing process safer and more efficient and also assisting in inventory management. These devices are essentially repositories, or *pharmaceutical vending machines*, for medications that will be dispensed directly from a patient care area. A variety of manufacturers of automated dispensing devices are in the market today—the Pyxis Medstation®, Meditrol®, Omnicell®, and SureMed® are some examples.

These machines are generally networked via a dedicated computer file server within the facility. They allow both unit-dose and bulk pharmaceuticals to be stocked securely on a given patient care unit location. Each unit's inventory is configurable and allows for variation and flexibility from device to device depending on its location. The machines are capable of tracking perpetual inventory at the product level. They also limit access to authorized personnel, record the identities of those who access inventory, and record how much was removed for each patient. A useful feature in many of these systems allows pharmacy personnel to generate automatically a fill-list of what needs to be replenished based on a par-level system. In essence, the nursing and medical personnel who use these automated dispensing devices have a computerized inventory and billing system that the pharmacy staff manages. Medications used to restock these devices may be taken from the pharmacy's main inventory, or a separate purchase order may be executed periodically for each device.

Regardless of the inventory system used, pharmacy technicians are vital contributors. The pharmacy technician may frequently identify changes in use or prescription patterns of pharmaceuticals. Examples might include high use of asthmatic medications (i.e., epinephrine, albuterol, or inhaled steroids) by the emergency department or various clinics, high doses of a particular antibiotic (e.g., chloramphenicol or liposomal amphotericin b) for a seriously ill patient who is likely to be hospitalized for an extended period, or high-dose opioid use by one or more oncology patients. Alerting purchasing staff to orders for unusual amounts of medications helps avoid out-of-stock situations and facilitates optimal inventory management.

Drug Recalls

A manufacturer or the Food and Drug Administration (FDA) will occasionally recall pharmaceuticals for such reasons as mislabeling, contamination, lack of potency, lack of adherence to good manufacturing practices, or other situations that may present a significant risk to public health. It is imperative that a pharmacy have a system for rapid removal of any recalled products including notification of patients if this is indicated.

Drug Shortages

Occasionally, manufacturers will be unable to supply a pharmaceutical because of various supply and demand situations. These situations may involve the inability to obtain raw materials, manufacturing difficulties related to equipment failure, or simply an inability to produce sufficient quantities to stay ahead of market demand. Although unfortunate, it is a reality that must be dealt with to avoid compromising patient care. As with drug recalls, the pharmacist in charge should be notified so he or she may communicate drug shortages and recommend alternative therapies to prescribers.

Ordering and Borrowing Pharmaceuticals

Pharmaceutical Purchasing Groups

Most health-system pharmacies are members of a group purchasing organization (GPO). Health systems and hospitals join together in a purchasing group to leverage their buying power and take advantage of lower prices manufacturers offer to large groups that can guarantee a significant volume of orders over long periods of time (typically 1 to 2 years). Retail chain pharmacies are also able to negotiate better pricing on the basis of volume. Contracts may involve sole-source or multisource products. Sole-source products are products available from only one manufacturer, whereas multisource products (frequently termed *generic* products) are available from numerous manufacturers. Sole-source products may be produced by only one manufacturer; however, they may be included in what is known as a *competitive market basket* (e.g., proton-pump-inhibitors, such as omeprazole and lansoprazole) when there are competing brand-name products on the market.

GPOs negotiate purchasing contracts that are mutually favorable to members of the group and to manufacturers. In addition to lower prices, pharmacies benefit from reduced time staff spent establishing and managing purchasing contracts with product vendors. A GPO guarantees the price for pharmaceuticals over the established contract period, which may be 1 or more years. With the purchase price predetermined, the pharmacy can order the product directly from the manufacturer or from a wholesale supplier. Occasionally, manufacturers are unable to supply a given product that the pharmacy is buying on contract. The pharmacy may then have to buy or substitute a competing product not on contract at a higher cost. Most purchasing contracts will include language to protect the pharmacy from incurring additional expenses in this event. Generally, the manufacturer will be liable to rebate the difference in cost back to the pharmacy. Therefore, it is important for the pharmacy technician to document any off-contract purchases and share them with the pharmacist in charge for reconciliation with the contracted vendor.

Direct Purchasing

Direct purchasing from a manufacturer involves the execution of a purchase order between the pharmacy and the manufacturer. The advantages of direct purchasing include not having to pay handling fees to a third-party wholesaler, the ability to order on an infrequent basis (e.g., once a month), and a less demanding system for monitoring inventory. Some disadvantages include the need for a large storage capacity; a large amount of cash invested in inventory; the complication of the pharmacy's return/credit process; and staff resources required in the pharmacy and accounts payable department to prepare, process, and pay purchase orders to more companies. Other

disadvantages have to do with the likelihood that the manufacturer's warehouse is not located near the pharmacy. The manufacturers depend on shipping firms to ship products reliably; however, delivery is often unpredictable or not available on weekends, and there may be delays in delivery.

For most pharmacies, the disadvantages of direct ordering outweigh the advantages. As a result, most pharmacies primarily purchase through a drug wholesaler. There are, however, some drugs that can only be purchased directly from the manufacturers. These products generally require unique control or storage conditions. Consequently, most pharmacies will have a combination of direct purchases from manufacturers and purchases from drug wholesalers.

Drug Wholesaler Purchasing/Prime Vendor Purchasing

Purchasing from a drug wholesaler permits the acquisition of drug products from different manufacturers through a single vendor. When a health-system pharmacy agrees to purchase the majority (90 to 95 percent) of its pharmaceuticals from a single wholesale company, a prime vendor arrangement is established, and, customarily, a contract between the pharmacy and the drug wholesaler is developed. Usually, the wholesaler agrees to deliver at least 95 to 98 percent of the items on schedule and offers 24-hour/7-day-per-week emergency service. The wholesaler also provides the pharmacy with electronic order entry or receiving devices, a computer system for ordering, bar-coded shelf stickers, and a printer for order confirmation printouts. It may also offer a highly competitive discount (minus 1 to 2 percent) below product cost and contract pricing and competitive alternate contract pricing. Some wholesalers will offer even larger discounts to pharmacies that may prefer a prepayment arrangement. In these situations, the wholesaler monitors the aggregate purchases of the pharmacy (e.g., a rolling 3-month average) and bills the pharmacy this amount in advance (prepayment). This arrangement creates larger cash flow and investment capital for the wholesaler while saving the pharmacy money on its pharmaceutical purchases.

These wholesaler services make the establishment of a prime vendor contract appealing and result in the following advantages: more timely ordering and delivery, less time spent creating purchase orders, fewer inventory carrying costs, less documentation, computer-generated lists of pharmaceuticals purchased, and overall simplification of the credit and return process. Purchasing through a prime vendor customarily allows for drugs to be received shortly before use, supporting the just-in-time ordering philosophy mentioned earlier in this chapter. Purchasing from a wholesaler is thus a highly efficient and cost-effective approach toward pharmaceutical purchasing and inventory management.

Borrowing Pharmaceuticals

No matter how effective a purchasing system is, the pharmacy occasionally must borrow drugs from other pharmacies. Most pharmacies have policies and procedures addressing this situation. Borrowing or loaning drugs between pharmacies is usually restricted to emergency situations and limited to authorized staff. Borrowing is also limited to products that are commercially available, thus eliminating such items as compounded products or investigational medications. Most pharmacies have developed forms to document and track merchandise that is borrowed or loaned (see **Figure 2-5**). These forms also help staff document the details necessary for error-free transactions.

The pharmacy's borrow and loan policies and procedures should provide detailed directions on how to borrow and loan products, which products may be borrowed or loaned, sources for them, and reconciliation of borrow-loan transactions (the payback process). Securing the borrowed item may require the use of a transport or courier service or may include the use of security staff or other designated personnel. This information is vital for pharmacy technicians to understand so they can fulfill their responsibility when borrowing and loaning products.

Products Requring Special Handling

Most pharmaceuticals, with the exception of controlled substances, investigational drugs, compounded prod-

ucts, repackaged drugs, and drug samples, will be handled and processed in the inventorying and purchasing systems described above.

Controlled Substances

Controlled substances have specific ordering, receiving, storage, dispensing, inventory, record-keeping, return, waste, and disposal requirements established under the law. The *Pharmacist's Manual: An Informational Outline of the Controlled Substances Act of 1970* and the *ASHP Technical Assistance Bulletin on Institutional Use of Controlled Substances* provide detailed information on the specific handling requirements for controlled substances.

The pharmacy technician should know two principles regarding controlled substances: (1) Ordering and receiving Schedule II controlled substances requires special order forms and additional time (1 to 3 days), and (2) these substances are inventoried and tracked continuously. This type of inventory method is referred to as a perpetual inventory process, whereby each dose or packaged unit, such as a tablet, vial, or ml of fluid volume, is accounted for at all times. In some pharmacies, pharmacy technicians work with pharmacists to manage inventory and order, dispense, store, and control narcotics and other controlled substances.

Investigational Drugs

Investigational drugs also require special ordering, inventorying, and handling procedures. Generally, the use of investigational drugs is categorized into two distinct areas: (1) investigational drugs used in a formal protocol that was approved by the institution or (2) investigational drugs used for a single patient on a one-time basis that has been authorized by the manufacturer and the FDA. In both cases, the physician may be responsible for the ordering and the pharmacy staff handles the inventory management of the investigational drug. Some pharmacies associated with academic affiliations or institutions conducting clinical research may have formally organized Investigational Drug Services managed by a pharmacist principally dedicated to pharmaceutical research activities. In these cases, the investigational drug service pharmacist may be responsible for the ordering, dispensing, and inventory management of investigational drugs according to the research protocol. Pharmacy technicians often prepare or handle investigational drugs and participate in the required perpetual inventory record-keeping system.

Community Pharmacy
555-3779

Borrowed   Lent
  From: _____   To: _____
Drug: _____
Amount: _____
              (# of vials, tablets, etc. and bulk or unit dose packaging)
Date:_____ By: _____

****

Date ordered:_____From: _____ By: _____
Date returned:_____ By: _____
Date in Loan Book:_____ By: _____
Value: $_____

Figure 2-5. Borrow/Loan Form

Again, it is important for pharmacy technicians to learn the department procedures for investigational drugs and to be competent in the handling, storage, dispensing, and inventory systems involved.

Compounded Products

Compounded pharmaceuticals are another type of product handled by pharmacy personnel. Unlike drugs ordered from an outside source, compounded products are extemporaneously prepared in the pharmacy as indicated by scientific compounding formulas. These products may include oral liquids, topical preparations, solid dosage forms, and sterile products.

The use of these products requires that prescribing patterns and expiration dates be monitored closely. Compounded products typically have short expiration dates, ranging from days to months. Because pharmacy technicians are likely to identify usage patterns and determine stock and product needs, procedures for monitoring patient use, product expiration dates, and additional stock needs must be well known and adhered to by technicians to prevent stock shortages. Specific pharmacy technicians may initiate compounding activities, but this may vary according to departmental procedures.

Repackaged Pharmaceuticals

Although manufacturers supply many drugs in a prepackaged unit-dose form, the pharmacy staff is responsible for packaging some products. These items are generally unit-dose tablets and capsules, unit-dose oral liquids, and some bulk packages of oral solids and liquids. Each pharmacy establishes stocking mechanisms for these products and relies on pharmacy technicians to identify and respond to production and stock needs. Generally, designated technicians coordinate prepackaging activities, but some pharmacies may integrate repackaging with other pharmacy technician responsibilities. Knowledge of the pharmacy's procedures for repackaging is required to prevent disruptions in dispensing activities.

Medication Samples

The last products requiring special handling are medication samples. Traditional inventory management and handling practices do not work well with medication samples for two reasons. First, medication samples are not ordered by the pharmacy; the drug manufacturer usually provides them to physicians, upon request, free of charge. This often occurs without the pharmacy's knowledge. Second, samples are not usually dispensed by the pharmacy. These factors make it difficult to know whom to contact if a medication sample is recalled and to ensure that medication samples are not sold. Because of difficulties in controlling samples, organizations may allow samples to be stored and dispensed in ambulatory clinics only after the samples are registered with the pharmacy for tracking purposes. These difficult logistical and control factors have led many organizations to adopt policies that simply disallow medication samples altogether.

If your organization does allow medication samples, they will probably be stored outside the pharmacy, and pharmacy personnel will be required to register and inspect the stock. Pharmacy technicians are sometimes involved in inspecting medication sample storage units. These technicians are often responsible for determining if a sample is registered with the pharmacy, stored in acceptable quantities, labeled with an expiration date that has not been exceeded, and stored under acceptable conditions. Review your pharmacy's policies and procedures regarding medication samples to learn the role of the pharmacy technician. Many hospitals strive to maintain compliance with the standards of the Joint Commission on Accreditation of Healthcare Organizations (JCAHO). Its standards on medication management are intended to promote consistently safe practices related to the procurement, storage, dispensing, and administration of pharmaceuticals, and the use of sample drug products falls into this standard.

Proper Disposal and Return of Pharmaceuticals

Expired Pharmaceuticals

The most common reason drugs are returned to the manufacturer is because they have expired. The process for returning drugs in the original manufacturer packaging is relatively simple and not particularly time-consuming when done routinely. Returning expired products to the manufacturer or wholesaler prevents the inadvertent use of these products and enables the pharmacy to receive either full or partial credit for them. Some wholesalers limit credit given on returns of short-dated products. Generally, wholesalers will not give full credit on returns of products that will expire within 6 months. To return products, pharmacy personnel must complete the documentation required by the product's manufacturer or wholesaler and package the product for shipment. Many wholesalers have implemented electronic documentation systems to further simplify the return process. Technicians often perform these duties under the supervision of a pharmacist. Some pharmacies contract with an outside vendor that completes the documentation and coordinates the return of these products for a fee. In this case, the pharmacy technician need only assist the returned goods vendor with locating and packaging the expired pharmaceuticals.

Pharmaceuticals compounded or repackaged by the pharmacy cannot be returned and must be disposed of after they have expired. It is important to dispose of these products for safety reasons. Proper disposal prevents the use of subpotent products or products whose sterility can no longer be guaranteed. The precise procedure for disposal depends on the type and content of the product. Some products, such as expired repackaged solids, can be disposed of via the general trash removal system, while others, such as expired compounded cytotoxic products, must be disposed of according to hazardous waste removal procedures. Each pharmacy has detailed procedures for hazardous waste removal, and the pharmacy technician should be familiar with these procedures. Disposal of expired compounded or repackaged pharmaceuticals by the pharmacy technician should be completed under the supervision of the pharmacist.

Other products requiring disposal rather than return are chemicals used in the pharmacy laboratory. Most pharmacies stock a supply of chemical-grade products used in extemporaneous pharmaceutical compounding. Examples of chemical products include sodium benzoate or sodium citrate (preservatives), lactose or talc (excipients), buffers, and active ingredients, such as hydrocortisone, triamcinolone, neomycin, or lidocaine powders. When such products expire, they should be disposed of in accordance with the pharmacy's hazardous waste procedures.

Expired controlled substances are disposed of in a unique way. These products may not be returned to the manufacturer or wholesaler for credit. They must be destroyed, and the destruction must be documented to the satisfaction of the Drug Enforcement Administration (DEA). The DEA provides a form, titled "Registrant's Inventory of Drugs Surrendered" (Form 41), for recording the disposal of expired controlled substances (see **Figure 2-6**). Ideally, the actual disposal of expired controlled substances should be completed by a company sanctioned by the DEA or by a representative of the state board of pharmacy. In other cases,

the DEA may allow the destruction of controlled substances by a pharmacy, provided an appropriate witness process is followed and documented. The DEA form for disposal of controlled substances should be completed properly and submitted to the DEA immediately after the disposal has occurred. A DEA representative signs a copy of the record of disposal form and returns it to the pharmacy, where it is kept on file. Previously, the DEA allowed for shipment of expired controlled substances and the completed disposal form to the regional DEA office, but this practice is no longer permitted.

The use and disposition of investigational drugs must also be documented carefully. Expired investigational drugs should be returned to the manufacturer or sponsor of an investigational drug study according to the instructions they provide. The pharmacy technician may be responsible, under the supervision of the pharmacist, for documenting, packaging, and shipping the expired investigational agents. Investigational drug products that expire because of product instability or sterility issues should never be discarded. These doses should be retained with the investigational drug stock and be clearly marked as expired drug products, since the investigational study sponsor will need to review and account for all expired investigational drug products.

Pharmaceuticals that need to be returned because of an ordering error require authorization from the original supplier and the appropriate forms. The Prescription Drug Marketing Act mandates that pharmacies retain the authorization and retention records of returned pharmaceuticals in order to prevent diversion of pharmaceuticals. The pharmacy technician must be familiar with pharmacy procedures for returning medications to a supplier. Typically, a pharmacy will have a process for returning misordered medications to the prime drug wholesaler on a routine basis. This prevents the need to store overstocked or misordered products in the pharmacy. The pharmacy technician may be responsible for relevant documentation, filing of paperwork, and the packaging of returned products under the supervision of the pharmacist.

Medical Devices and Associated Supplies

Many of the inventory management processes discussed in relation to pharmaceuticals also hold true for medical devices and associated supplies. One unique feature of the medical device business, however, is that some of the equipment is provided to patients on a rental or lease agreement rather than an outright

| OMB Approval
No. 1117 - 0007 | U. S. Department of Justice / Drug Enforcement Administration
REGISTRANTS INVENTORY OF DRUGS SURRENDERED | PACKAGE NO. |

The following schedule is an inventory of controlled substances which is hereby surrendered to you for proper disposition.

FROM: *(Include Name, Street, City, State and ZIP Code in space provided below.)*

Signature of applicant or authorized agent

Registrant's DEA Number

Registrant's Telephone Number

NOTE: CERTIFIED MAIL (Return Receipt Requested) IS REQUIRED FOR SHIPMENTS OF DRUGS VIA U.S. POSTAL SERVICE. See instructions on reverse (page 2) of form.

NAME OF DRUG OR PREPARATION Registrants will fill in Columns 1,2,3, and 4 ONLY.	Number of Con-tainers	CONTENTS (Number of grams, tablets, ounces or other units per con-tainer)	Con-trolled Sub-stance Con-tent, (Each Unit)	FOR DEA USE ONLY		
				DISPOSITION	QUANTITY	
					GMS.	MGS.
1	2	3	4	5	6	7
1						
2						
3						
4						
5						
6						
7						
8						
9						
10						
11						
12						
13						
14						
15						
16						

FORM DEA-41 (9-01)   Previous edition dated **6-86** is usable.   *See instructions on reverse (page 2) of form.*

Figure 2-6. DEA Form 41 (Registrants Inventory of Drugs Surrendered)

Source: Drug Enforcement Administration http://www.deadiversion.usdoj.gov/21cfr_reports/surrend/41/41_blank.pdf

purchase. In these instances, it is important that returned equipment be properly processed before being rented or leased to the next patient. Processing always includes a thorough cleaning with an approved disinfecting agent and may include sterilization of parts that come into direct contact with the patient. Between patient uses or periodically according to the manufacturer's recommendations, equipment will also undergo a biomedical review to make sure it is in proper working order, has had indicated preventive maintenance performed, and is safe for patient use. Biomedical reviews are also performed in response to reported malfunctions.

It is important to ensure that patients have the proper supplies to use with any medical equipment. Patients often need assistance in completing forms to ensure proper reimbursement related to medical devices and supplies.

It is also often necessary for a pharmacy offering medical supplies and equipment to employ staff with special training and even certifications in the fitting and use of the devices. These staff members, who may be technicians, generally assist patients in choosing the appropriate device upon a physician recommendation, help the patients ensure proper fit and match supplies to the particular device, and help educate the patients on the use of their equipment. They may also be responsible for some of the cleaning and preventive maintenance on reusable equipment.

Summary

The movement of pharmaceuticals into and out of the pharmacy requires an organized, systematic, and cooperative approach. The pharmacy technician plays a vital role in maintaining the functionality of these systems as the medication is ultimately used to provide pharmaceutical care. Pharmacy technicians' familiarity with product conditions and uses positions them to identify quality and care issues that can strengthen the purchasing and inventory control system.

Suggested Reading

From *Manual for Pharmacy Technicians*, 3rd ed.

Drug Distribution Processes: See Chapter 2—Ambulatory Care Pharmacy Practice, Chapter 3—Institutional Pharmacy Practice, and Chapter 4—Home Care Pharmacy Practice.

Inventory Procedures: See Chapter 16—Purchasing and Inventory Control and Chapter 6—Pharmacy Law.

Compounding and Repackaging Requirements: See Chapter 13—Nonsterile Compounding and Repackaging.

Self-Assessment Questions

1. The decision to add a drug to a hospital's formulary should always be based on which drug is cheapest to purchase.
   a. True
   b. False

2. Which of the following is *not* a part of the normal receiving process for pharmaceuticals received from the drug wholesaler?
   a. Complete the required documentation on any investigational drugs included in the shipment.
   b. Complete the required documentation on any controlled substances included in the shipment.
   c. Verify that the box count is correct and that there are no damaged packages
   d. Verify that all items are received and that the inventory is not expired or close to expiration.
   e. Sign and date the purchase order.

3. Provide the appropriate USP definition for each temperature.
   a. > 40° C
   b. 20° to 25° C
   c. -25° to -10° C
   d. 2° to 8° C
   e. Prevailing temperature in the work area

4. Which statement is *true* regarding the placement of medications on the shelves to prevent medication errors?
   a. Generic label drugs should not be placed near the brand-name product.
   b. Look-alike drugs may be mistaken for each other and should be stored in different locations when possible.
   c. Different strengths of the same medication should never be stored next to each other because the wrong strength might be picked.
   d. The prominent placement of company logos does not contribute to medication errors and is not a factor in determining shelf placement.
   e. All of the above

5. The Pareto ABC system relies on the premise that managing 20 percent of your inventory will cover 80 percent of your costs (the 80/20 rule).
   a. True
   b. False

6. Calculate the inventory turnover rate if the pharmacy's annual purchases were $4,866,255 and the inventory as of December 31 was $286,423.
   a. 22 times
   b. 14 times
   c. 19 times
   d. 17 times
   e. 10 times

7. Why may the FDA direct a manufacturer to recall a pharmaceutical?
   a. because of contamination
   b. because of lack of potency
   c. because of lack of adherence to good manufacturing practices
   d. because of any situation that may present a significant risk to public health
   e. all of the above

8. Which of the following is *not* an example of a drug that requires special handling during receiving in the pharmacy?
   a. samples
   b. controlled substances
   c. injectables
   d. investigational drugs
   e. compounded or repackaged items

9. The DEA Form 41 is required when controlled substances are expired and need to be disposed of.
   a. True
   b. False

10. Reusable medical devices must be
    a. cleaned between patient uses
    b. checked between uses to ensure that they are functioning properly
    c. maintained with all manufacturer-recommended preventive maintenance
    d. tested for proper function in response to any report of malfunction
    e. all of the above

Self-Assessment Answers

1. b
2. a
3. excessive heat; controlled room temperature; freezer; refrigerated; room temperature
4. b
5. a
6. d
7. e
8. c
9. a
10. e

Pharmacy Operations

3

Policies and Procedures

Policies and procedures (P&P) are documents that provide guidance about expectations of the behavior of employees of the hospital, business, or pharmacy department. General P&P cover areas such as hiring requirements and employee benefits. Pharmacy P&P cover issues concerning the delivery of efficient, quality drug therapy, including the following:

- correct aseptic (sterile) technique when compounding intravenous (IV) admixtures
- good compounding practices
- repackaging processes
- monitoring patients for drug allergies
- proper handling of cancer chemotherapeutic agents
- distribution and control of all drugs used in the organization
- procedures for ensuring that patients receive the correct drugs
- use of investigational (experimental) drugs
- management of toxic or dangerous drugs
- provision of pharmacy services in the event of a disaster
- identification of medications brought into the organization by patients
- management of drug expenditures and the pharmacy budget
- staffing levels
- identification of prescription forgeries and theft prevention strategies
- billing procedures and maintenance of customer accounts
- inventory control and maintenance procedures
- management of medical equipment

Many accrediting organizations, such as the Joint Commission on Accreditation of Healthcare Organizations (JCAHO), and professional organizations, such as the American Society of Health-System Pharmacists (ASHP), require that pharmacy departments develop and maintain P&P manuals. Pharmacy department P&P are developed by the director of pharmacy or the pharmacist-in-charge or owner in a retail establishment (or by corporate headquarters for a chain store). These documents are generally revised and updated annually and are compiled in a readily available manual or kept available online for easy access by all employees.

Learning Objectives

After completing this chapter, the technician should be able to

1. Give examples of policies and procedures relating to the practice of pharmacy.

2. Differentiate between quality control and continuous quality improvement mechanisms.

3. List the elements required by federal law to be on a prescription label.

4. List exemptions to the Poison Prevention Packaging Act.

5. Discuss special handling requirements for controlled substances.

6. State the intent of the Omnibus Budget Reconciliation Act of 1990 (OBRA 90) and describe the requirements it mandates.

7. State the intent of the Health Insurance Portability and Accountability Act of 1996 (HIPAA) and describe the requirements it mandates.

8. Discuss pharmacy record-keeping requirements.

9. Describe the correct procedures for cleaning and maintaining equipment used in compounding.

Quality Assurance Mechanisms

Quality control and continuous quality improvement (CQI) programs are also required by many of the accrediting agencies, such as the JCAHO and the Centers for Medicare and Medicaid Services (CMS; formerly the Health Care Financing Administration, or HCFA). Quality improvement is good practice, even if it is not required by regulatory oversight. Improving the efficiency and accuracy of our medication use systems—both inpatient and outpatient—means healthier and happier patients and customers and decreased overall health care costs. The following are just a few examples of quality control and quality improvement activities:

- completing refrigerator temperature logs
- documenting inspections of nursing units and other medication stock areas
- decreasing legibility errors by working with local physicians to provide electronic prescription transmission
- improving medication turnaround time in the hospital by automating dispensing
- decreasing wrong-drug/wrong-patient errors through the use of bar-code identification systems
- updating patient files at each prescription encounter to ensure that patient information is correct

Quality can be ensured through the use of quality control and through continuous quality improvement methods.

Quality Control

Quality control is a set of procedures followed during the manufacturing of a product or provision of a service to ensure that the end product or service meets or exceeds specified standards. Checks and balances usually occur at critical points in the process. The start of any quality control program requires complete written procedures and training for all staff members involved in that procedure. Although quality control identifies and prevents errors or defects, it does not always identify or correct the underlying cause.

Continuous Quality Improvement

CQI is a scientific and systematic process involving monitoring, evaluating, and identifying problems and developing and measuring the impact of the improvement strategies. It requires that decisions be based on data. Various tools have been used to identify problems, assist in the data collection, and analyze the data.

Workflow diagrams, run charts (which track patterns and trends over a period of time), and Pareto analysis (the 80/20 rule) are examples of tools used in CQI.

Compliance with Federal and State Law

Prescription Label Requirements

The Food, Drug and Cosmetic Act (FDCA) requires that all retail prescription labels have the following information: name and address of pharmacy; prescription number; date of prescription filling or refilling; name of prescriber; name of patient; directions for use; and cautionary statement (as indicated on the prescription). Medication orders in long-term care facilities and hospitals are different from retail prescriptions; therefore, the labels do not require the same information. Labels on medicines in long-term care facilities or hospitals may not include quantity dispensed, cautionary statements, original filling date, prescriber's name, or even the name and address of the pharmacy. Most states have rules for what must appear on prescription or medication order labels. Therefore, the technician should review the state's rules regarding labeling.

Prescription Refill Requirements

A prescription can usually be refilled as many times as the prescriber indicates on the prescription, within a time period determined by the state. This time period is usually 1 year from the date the prescription was written. If the number of refills does not appear on the prescription, it is assumed that refills are not authorized.

When a prescription is refilled, state law usually requires that a note be made on the back of the prescription indicating the quantity dispensed, the date dispensed, and the pharmacist's initials. This information is now typically kept electronically.

Patients who do not have refills on a prescription may request that the pharmacist ask the prescriber to authorize refills. An emergency supply of medication, usually not more than a 72-hour supply, may be dispensed to a patient if the pharmacist is unable to obtain refill authorization and determines that the patient may suffer harm if a lapse in therapy occurs.

Poison Prevention Packaging Act

The Poison Prevention Packaging Act was enacted to reduce the number of poisonings in children from drugs and chemicals. It has been remarkably successful.

The law requires that all prescriptions and most over-the-counter drugs be dispensed in containers with child-resistant closures, unless the drug or container falls under one of the many exceptions. These child-resistant prescription containers cannot be reused for refills. This law usually applies to retail settings. It does not apply to the dispensing of prescriptions to inpatients in long-term care facilities or hospitals, but it does apply to prescriptions dispensed to those patients upon discharge. Therefore, when filling a prescription for a patient who is being discharged from the institution to return home, the drug must be dispensed in a container with a child-resistant closure.

Some drugs, such as nitroglycerin, oral contraceptives, and other drugs packaged for patient use by the manufacturer (such as prepackaged methylprednisolone), do not require the child-resistant container. The list, with exceptions, of drugs that require safety closures is available from the U.S. Consumer Product Safety Commission's Web site, http://www.cpsc.gov/CPSCPUB/PUBS/384.pdf.

Because many patients do not have children at home or may have a disease that impairs their ability to open child-resistant containers, the patient, caregiver, or physician may request that the prescription be dispensed in a non-child-resistant container. Federal law does not require a written request to have the prescription dispensed in a non-child-resistant container. However, physicians who make this request must do so on a patient-by-patient basis and not in the form of a blanket request for all or a group of patients.

Controlled Substance Regulations

The Federal Controlled Substance Act was enacted to protect the public by controlling the flow of dangerous drugs into the community. The United States Department of Justice Drug Enforcement Agency (DEA) takes responsibility for vigilance over the distribution of these drugs in research, institutions, and the community. This agency plays an important role in creating the rules that govern the practice of pharmacy.

Drugs that are watched by the DEA are called *controlled substances*. Controlled substances are divided into five categories, or schedules. Schedule I drugs are substances with a high abuse potential and no legitimate medical purpose. Schedule II drugs are those with high abuse potential and a recognized medical purpose. Schedules III, IV, and V drugs have legitimate medical purpose but less abuse potential. For all practical

purposes, Schedules III, IV, and V drugs are treated the same from a regulatory perspective.

To order a prescription for a controlled substance, the prescriber must be registered with the Department of Justice and be issued a DEA registration number. Similarly, to dispense a controlled substance, a pharmacy must have a DEA registration number.

Schedules of Controlled Substances

Schedule II. Some examples of single-entity Schedule II narcotics include morphine, codeine, hydrocodone, and opium. Other Schedule II narcotic substances and their common name-brand products include hydromorphone (Dilaudid®), methadone (Dolophine®), meperidine (Demerol®), oxycodone (Percodan®), and fentanyl (Sublimaze®). Some examples of Schedule II stimulants include amphetamine (Dexedrine®, Adderall®), methamphetamine (Desoxyn®), and methylphenidate (Ritalin®). Other Schedule II substances include cocaine, amobarbital, glutethimide, pentobarbital, and secobarbital.

Schedule III. Some examples of Schedule III narcotics include products containing less than 15 milligrams of hydrocodone per dosage unit (Vicodin®, Lorcet®, Tussionex®) and products containing not more than 90 milligrams of codeine per dosage unit (codeine with acetaminophen, aspirin, or ibuprofen). Other Schedule III substances include anabolic steroids; benzphetamine (Didrex®); phendimetrazine; and any compound, mixture, preparation, or suppository dosage form containing amobarbital, secobarbital, pentobarbital, dronabinol (Marinol®), or ketamine.

Schedule IV. The substances in this schedule have an abuse potential less than those in Schedule III and more than those in Schedule V. Some examples of Schedule IV narcotics include propoxyphene (Darvon®), butorphanol (Stadol®), and pentazocine (Talwin-NX®). The following benzodiazepine substances are also found in Schedule IV: alprazolam (Xanax®), clonazepam (Klonopin®), clorazepate (Tranxene®), diazepam (Valium®), flurazepam (Dalmane®), halazepam (Paxipam®), lorazepam (Ativan®), midazolam (Versed®), oxazepam (Serax®), prazepam (Centrax®), temazepam (Restoril®), triazolam (Halcion®), and quazepam (Doral®). Other Schedule IV substances include barbital, phenobarbital, chloral hydrate, ethchlorvynol (Placidyl®), chlordiazepoxide (Librium®), ethinamate, meprobamate, paraldehyde, methohexital, phentermine, diethylpropion, pemoline (Cylert®), mazindol (Sanorex®), and sibutramine (Meridia®).

Schedule V. The substances in this schedule have an abuse potential less than those in Schedule IV and consist primarily of preparations containing limited quantities of certain narcotic and stimulant drugs, generally for antitussive, antidiarrheal, or analgesic purposes. Some examples are cough preparations containing not more than 200 milligrams of codeine per 100 milliliters or per 100 grams (Robitussin AC®, Phenergan with Codeine®) and buprenorphine (Buprenex®).

List I Chemicals. In addition to Schedules I through V controlled substances, the DEA monitors List I and List II chemicals. These are chemicals that can be used in the synthesis of other chemicals that are controlled substances. The pharmacy must account for List I and List II chemicals. Three common List I chemicals are ephedrine, phenylpropanolamine (PPA), and pseudoephedrine. The use of these chemicals in compounding may have to be reported to the DEA, depending on a state's rules.

States also will place certain drugs into a schedule. Occasionally, a conflict arises when a state and the federal government do not agree on which schedule a drug should be. If such a conflict arises, the stricter scheduling will apply.

Ordering Controlled Substances

Schedule I and II Substances

Schedule I and II controlled substances are ordered with a DEA form 222 (Official Order Form). This Official Order Form is required for each distribution, purchase, or transfer of a Schedule II controlled substance from one DEA registrant to another (i.e., wholesaler to pharmacy, pharmacy to pharmacy, or pharmacy to physician). These forms are to be used only when purchasing, distributing, or transferring drugs that are federally Schedule I or II.

Completing Official Order Forms

Anyone can enter information on the 222 form. That person must fill in the number of packages, the size of the packages, and the name of the item. It's also a good idea to enter the National Drug Code (NDC) of the item being ordered. However, each Official Order Form can only be signed and dated by the person who signed the pharmacy registration application or by a person who has been given a power of attorney to sign it.

The 222 form is a triplicate form. The top page goes to the supplier of the drugs, the middle page is

sent to the DEA by the supplier of the drugs, and the last page stays with the purchaser. When the items are received, the pharmacist must document on the purchaser's copy (copy 3) the actual number of packages received and the date received. Official Order Forms must be maintained separately from the purchaser's (pharmacy's) other business records. The pharmacy may attach its copy to a copy of the supplier's invoice for that order.

The Code of Federal Regulations ([2004] 21 CFR1305) requires that the Official Order Form be "complete, legible, and properly prepared, with no signs of alteration, erasure or change of any description." A supplier may refuse to accept an order for any of these reasons. However, DEA has acknowledged that a supplier may accept some minor changes or alterations. For example, suppliers may correct Official Order Forms that have minor errors, that lack inconsequential information, or that have an incorrect date unintentionally annotated by the purchaser.

If the supplier refuses to fill an order, the Official Order Form (copies 1 and 2) must be returned to the purchaser with a statement explaining the reason the order was refused.

DEA policy does not prohibit the substitution of identical products differing in packaging size from those initially ordered, provided the actual quantity received does not exceed the amount initially ordered. For example, if a pharmacy orders 500 secobarbital capsules, the distributor may ship either one bottle of 500 capsules or five bottles of 100 capsules.

Power of Attorney to Sign an Official Order Form

Any registrant (e.g., a pharmacy, physician) may authorize one or more individuals, including technicians, to obtain and execute Official Order Forms by granting a power of attorney to each such individual. The person who signed the most recent application for registration or renewal registration, as well as the individual being authorized to obtain and execute Official Order Forms, must sign the power of attorney.

The person who granted the power of attorney may revoke it at any time. The power of attorney should be filed in the pharmacy along with the completed Official Order Forms and should be readily retrievable. The power of attorney is not submitted to the DEA.

Lost or Stolen Order Forms

When the pharmacist has not received a shipment of controlled substances, he or she should first contact the supplier to determine whether the original DEA form

222 was received. If the original order form has been lost or stolen, the pharmacist must complete a second order form so the supplier can fill the original order. The pharmacist must also prepare a statement that includes the first order form's serial number and date, verify that the drugs ordered were never received, and attach a copy of the statement to the second order form that is sent to the supplier. The pharmacist must keep a copy of the statement with copy 3 from the first and second order forms. Upon discovery of the loss or theft of unused order forms, a pharmacy must immediately report the loss to the nearest DEA Diversion Field Office and provide the serial numbers of each lost or stolen order form. If an entire book or multiple books of order forms are lost or stolen and the serial numbers of the missing forms cannot be identified, then the pharmacist must report the approximate date of issuance (in lieu of the serial numbers) to the DEA. If an unused order form reported stolen or lost is later recovered or found, the pharmacy must immediately notify the nearest DEA Diversion Field Office.

Schedule III–V Substances

The DEA registrant (pharmacy) must keep a receipt (i.e., invoice or packing slip) and record on it the date the drugs were received and confirm that the order is accurate. These receipts must be maintained in a readily retrievable manner for inspection by the DEA.

Counseling Requirements

The Omnibus Reconciliation Act of 1990 (OBRA 90) required states that receive federal funding to create programs to improve the quality of pharmaceutical care and save money by educating patients on the proper use of drugs. The program required pharmacists to obtain certain information from the patient, including personal identifying information, disease state, medication allergies, and other information that would be important for determining proper drug therapy. This federal program targeted only Medicaid and Medicare patients, but most states expanded it to include all patients.

Although most states require the pharmacist to provide the counseling, the pharmacy technician's role in this program is important in obtaining information from the patient. The extent of the technician's involvement in gathering information from the patient will be directly related to his or her ability to communicate effectively with patients and knowledge of disease and pharmaceutical terminology.

OBRA 90 further mandated that pharmacists provide counseling for individuals or their caregivers. The pharmacist or a designee must extend an offer for medication counseling to the patient. The offer may be written or oral. The pharmacist must always perform the actual counseling session. The patient may decline counseling, and, if so, this should be documented.

OBRA 90 and most state counseling regulations require that the following eight areas be covered in patient counseling:

- the name and description of the medication
- the route of administration, dosage, and dosage form
- special directions and precautions for preparation, administration, and use by the patient
- common severe side effects, adverse effects, interactions, and therapeutic contraindications
- techniques for self-monitoring therapy
- proper storage
- prescription refill information
- action to be taken in the case of a missed dose

The Health Insurance Portability and Accountability Act of 1996

The Health Insurance Portability and Accountability Act of 1996 (HIPAA) has strengthened patient privacy rights. While this was not the only purpose of the law, the pharmacy's role in maintaining confidentiality has also increased. Patient records must be guarded from disclosure to unauthorized individuals and companies. Pharmacy employees are prohibited from discussing a patient's medical history except for purposes relevant to the patient's care. All written information concerning a patient should be discarded in such a manner as to protect the patient's identity. Utilizing shredders or professional document disposal services is now common pharmacy practice. Pharmacy technicians should only discuss information regarding the patient's therapy so that unauthorized persons will not overhear such discussions. Technicians should also be aware that using overhead paging systems to announce a patient's name could undermine a patient's privacy. Most pharmacies will have policies and procedures in place to address the requirements of HIPAA.

Record-Keeping Requirements

The FDCA describes the records that pharmacists are required to keep. One of the main reasons pharmacists are required to record the receipt, disposition, and accountability of drugs is to ensure that the pharmacy can contact patients who received a drug that has been recalled.

Purchase invoices are records of drug receipt, prescriptions are records of drug disposition, and inventories provide a record of drugs in stock. Some type of written document should evidence any sales, disposals, returns, destruction, or theft of drugs. Rules vary as to the length of time records must be kept, but in general, it should not be less than 5 years. Some states may require longer storage of certain records.

Maintenance of Pharmacy Equipment

Cross-contamination resulting from microbes or drug product residue on equipment and work surfaces will not occur if written policies regarding cleaning and maintenance are followed and documented. Most automatic, mechanical, electronic, or other types of equipment have written programs for maintenance and cleaning to ensure proper performance. Technicians should familiarize themselves with these programs and document that these procedures have been completed as part of an ongoing quality assurance program. For example, laminar airflow hoods (LAHs) should be cleaned before use, compounding equipment should be inspected and maintained according to manufacturers' recommendations, and temperature control equipment should be monitored for temperature and be equipped with an alarm that sounds when the temperature exceeds predefined limits. All equipment maintenance should be completed on a schedule and documented.[1] Equipment cleaning, maintenance, and use should be recorded in individual equipment logs.

Nonsterile Compounding

All equipment and accessories used in compounding should be thoroughly cleaned after each use. Maintenance should be completed on the schedule recommended by the manufacturer and recorded. Weighing equipment should be certified at least annually. Guidelines for checking torsion balances can be found in pharmacy reference texts such as *Remington's Pharmaceutical Sciences*[2] or the *United States Pharmacopeia* and the *National Formulary*.[3]

Sterile Compounding

Sterile parenteral solutions must be kept free of living microorganisms, particulate matter, and pyrogens. This can be done by following several practices to maintain the sterile compounding area.

A sterile compounding area should be cleaned daily and segregated from normal pharmacy operations, patient specimens, nonessential equipment, and other materials that produce particles. Floors should be disinfected daily, and trash should be removed frequently. Stricter standards must be maintained if Risk Level II (batched solutions) or Risk Level III (sterile solutions from nonsterile ingredients) products are prepared in the area.

Laminar Airflow Hoods

The manufacturer's recommendations for proper operation and maintenance of LAHs should be followed. LAHs should be tested by qualified personnel every 6 months, whenever the hood is moved, or if filter damage is suspected. Specific tests are used to certify airflow velocity and high-efficiency particulate air (HEPA) filter integrity. HEPA filters should be inspected every 6 months and have their pre-filters changed monthly.

When cleaning LAHs, the technician should work from the cleanest area (directly in front of the flow of air from the HEPA filter) to the dirtiest area (generally farthest from the HEPA filter and closest to room air). LAHs should be cleaned with water if soiled, and disinfected with 70 percent isopropyl alcohol before each session. Cleaning should be done periodically during use when the surface is soiled.

Any cleaning procedure should take into consideration what drugs have been mixed in the space. If toxic materials have been used in the LAH, proper protective equipment should be used during cleaning. Cleaning materials should be properly disposed of to protect others from exposure.

Automated Compounders

Equipment used inside the LAH must be cleaned daily according to the manufacturer's instructions. These systems also require routine maintenance and calibration to ensure accurate compounding measurements.

Repackaging Equipment

Equipment used in repackaging may provide a medium for cross-contamination. Like equipment used in compounding, it should be cleaned after each use.

Suggested Reading

From *Manual for Pharmacy Technicians,* 3rd ed.:

Policies and Procedures: See Chapter 1—Introduction to Pharmacy.

Law: See Chapter 6—Pharmacy Law.

Quality Assurance: See Chapter 3—Institutional Pharmacy Practice.

Equipment Care and Maintenance: See Chapter 13—Nonsterile Compounding and Repackaging and Chapter 14—Aseptic Technique, Sterile Compounding, and Intravenous Admixture Programs.

References

1. Schneider PJ, ed. Equipment for compounding sterile preparations. In: Compounding sterile preparations, 2nd ed. Buchanan EC, Schneider PJ, eds. Bethesda, MD: American Society of Health-System Pharmacists; 2005:27–34.

2. Gennaro AR, ed. Remington's pharmaceutical sciences, 18th ed. Easton, PA: Mack Publishing; 1990:1631, 1658, 1660.

3. The United States pharmacopeia, 22nd rev. ed., and the national formulary, 17th ed. Rockville, MD: The United States Pharmacopeial Convention; 1989.

Self-Assessment Questions

1. What topics do policies and procedures generally cover?
    a. steps to follow when making an IV solution
    b. how the pharmacy should respond in an emergency
    c. staffing levels for the pharmacy
    d. how drug distribution is done
    e. all of the above

2. Quality control programs make sure that processes are working the way they are expected to, whereas quality improvement programs strive to make processes work better than before.
    a. True
    b. False

3. If a patient is out of refills but needs the medication, which of the following is (are) true for the pharmacist?
    a. can dispense an emergency supply if the physician cannot be contacted
    b. cannot dispense an emergency supply without violating the law
    c. can call the physician to obtain refills for the patient
    d. can refill the prescription without calling the physician if it is obvious that the medication is supposed to be continued
    e. both a and c

4. Which of the following medications are exempt from the Poison Prevention Packaging Act?
    a. oral contraceptives
    b. nitroglycerin
    c. medications packaged for patient use by the manufacturer
    d. all of the above
    e. no drugs are exempt from this important safety legislation

5. Schedule I drugs have a high abuse potential and are only rarely used medically.
    a. True
    b. False

6. What does OBRA 90 require?
    a. that pharmacists make the offer to counsel
    b. that the offer to counsel be made in writing
    c. that the pharmacist include a number of elements in education, including what to do if a dose is missed
    d. that there be a minimum of two pharmacists on duty at all times so that one is available to do counseling
    e. that someone provide counseling, but that person can be a pharmacist or a technician—whoever is free at the time

7. The Health Insurance Portability and Accountability Act of 1996 strengthened patient privacy protection for health information.
    a. True
    b. False

8. Record retention rules vary by state, but the minimum amount of time most records should be retained is 7 years.
    a. True
    b. False

9. How should laminar airflow hoods be cleaned?
    a. with water and disinfected with 70 percent isopropyl alcohol
    b. from the dirtiest area to the cleanest
    c. always the same way regardless of what was last prepared in the hood
    d. both a and b
    e. none of the above

10. What should routine maintenance of the sterile compounding area include?
    a. LAH pre-filter should be changed monthly
    b. floor should be cleaned daily
    c. trash should be emptied frequently
    d. HEPA filter should be inspected every 6 months
    e. all of the above

Self-Assessment Answers

1. e
2. a
3. e
4. d
5. b
6. c
7. a
8. b
9. a
10. e

Pharmacy Calculations Review

This chapter reviews the fundamentals of calculations and how those calculations are applied in pharmacy. For additional review and practice problems, see Chapter 5, Pharmacy Calculation, in *Manual for Pharmacy Technicians,* third edition.

Review of Basic Mathematical Functions Involving Fractions

All fractions must be converted to a common denominator when adding and subtracting. When multiplying and dividing, however, this conversion is not necessary. When working with fractions, the answer should be expressed as the smallest reduced fraction (i.e., if the answer is 6/8, it should be reduced to 3/4).

Addition

The following steps are necessary to add these fractions: 3/4 + 7/8 + 1/4

1. Convert all fractions to common denominators:

   3/4 × 2/2 = 6/8

   1/4 × 2/2 = 2/8

2. Add: 6/8 + 7/8 + 2/8 = 15/8

3. Reduce to the smallest fraction:

   15/8 = 1 7/8

Subtraction

The following steps are necessary to subtract these fractions: 7/8 − 1/4

1. Convert the fractions to common denominators:

   1/4 × 2/2 = 2/8

2. Subtract: 7/8 − 2/8 = 5/8

Multiplication

The following steps are necessary to multiply these fractions: 1/6 × 2/3

When multiplying and dividing fractions, it is not necessary to convert to common denominators.

1. Multiply the numerators: 1 × 2 = 2

2. Multiply the denominators: 6 × 3 = 18

Learning Objectives

After completing this chapter, the technician should be able to

1. Perform basic mathematical functions involving fractions.

2. Convert easily among fractions, decimals, percentages, and mixed numbers.

3. Work with various measurement systems, including metric, apothecary, avoirdupois, and household, and convert measurements in one system to equivalent measurements in other systems.

4. Perform temperature conversions between centigrade and Fahrenheit.

5. Perform body surface area (BSA) and ideal body weight (IBW) calculations.

6. Perform pharmacy calculations involving ratio/proportion and concentration/dilution.

7. Perform dosage and flow-rate calculations.

8. Perform simple statistical calculations.

3. Express the answer as a fraction: 2/18
4. Reduce the fraction: 2/18 = 1/9

Division

The following steps are necessary to divide these fractions: 1/2 ÷ 1/4

Once again, it is not necessary to convert to common denominators.

To divide two fractions, the first fraction must be multiplied by the inverse (or reciprocal) of the second fraction.

1. Invert the second fraction: 1/4 becomes 4/1.
2. Multiply: 1/2 × 4/1 = 4/2
3. Reduce to lowest fraction: 4/2 = 2

Converting Fractions to Decimal Numbers

To convert a fraction to a decimal number, the numerator is simply divided by the denominator.

For example, 1/2 = 1 divided by 2 = 0.5

Converting Mixed Numbers to Decimal Numbers

The process of converting mixed numbers to decimal numbers involves the following two steps:

1. Write the mixed number as a fraction.

   Method: Multiply the whole number and the denominator of the fraction. Add the product (result) to the numerator of the fraction, keeping the same denominator.

   Example: [(2×4)+3]/4 = 2 times 4 plus 3 over 4 = 11/4

2. Divide the numerator by the denominator.

   Example: 11/4 = 11 divided by 4 = 2.75

An alternate method involves the following three steps:

1. Separate the whole number and the fraction.

   Example: 2 3/4 = 2 and 3/4

2. Convert the fraction to its decimal counterpart.

   Example: 3/4 = 3 divided by 4 = 0.75

3. Add the whole number to the decimal fraction.

   Example: 2 plus 0.75 = 2.75

Converting Decimal Numbers to Mixed Numbers or Fractions

The process of converting decimal numbers to mixed numbers involves the following two steps:

1. Write the decimal number over 1, dividing it by 1.

(Remember that dividing any number by 1 does not change the number.)

Example: 3.5 = 3.5/1

2. Move the decimal point in both the numerator and denominator an equal number of places to the right. The number of places the decimal point needs to be moved is determined by the number of digits following the decimal point in the numerator.

   Example: Because there is only one digit following the decimal point in *3.5*, move the decimal point one place to the right in both the numerator and the denominator: 3.5/1 = 35/10.

   The number will remain the same as long as the same steps are taken with the numerator and the denominator. Remember that the decimal point of a whole number always follows the last digit.

3. Simplify the fraction.

   Example: 35/10 = 7/2 = 3 1/2

Percentages

Percentage (%) means "by the hundred" or "in a hundred." Percents are just fractions, but fractions with a set denominator. The denominator is always one hundred (100).

   Example: "50%" means "50 in a hundred" or "50/100" or "1/2"

Converting Percentages to Fractions

To convert a percentage to a fraction, one would write the number preceding the percent sign over 100 and simplify the resulting fraction.

   Example: 25% = 25/100 = 1/4

Converting Fractions to Percentages

To convert a fraction to a percentage, one must take the following steps to convert the fraction to one in which the denominator is a hundred. This is easiest when the fraction is in the form of a decimal.

1. Write the fraction in its decimal form.

   Example: 3/4 = 3 divided by 4 = 0.75

2. Write the decimal over 1.

   Example: 0.75/1

3. To obtain 100 as the denominator, move the decimal point two places to the right. To avoid changing the value, move the decimal point two places to the right in the numerator as well.

Example: 0.75/1 = 75/100

4. Because we already know that "out of a hundred" or "divided by a hundred" is the same as percent, we can write 75/100 as 75%.

Concentration Expressed as a Percentage

Percent weight-in-weight (w/w) is the grams of a drug in 100 grams of the product.

Percent weight-in-volume (w/v) is the grams of a drug in 100 milliliters (ml) of the product.

Percent volume-in-volume (v/v) is the milliliters of drug in 100 ml of the product.

These concentration percentages will be discussed in detail a little later in this chapter.

Units of Measure

Metric System

The metric system is based on the decimal system, in which everything is measured in multiples or fractions of ten.

Standard Measures

The standard measure for length is the *meter*, the standard measure for weight is the *gram*, and the standard measure for volume is the *liter*.

Prefixes

The prefixes below are used to describe multiples or fractions of the standard measures for length, weight, and volume.

Latin prefixes

micro- (mc):	1/1,000,000	= 0.000001
milli- (m):	1/1,000	= 0.001
centi- (c):	1/100	= 0.01
deci- (d):	1/10	= 0.1

Latin prefixes denote fractions.

Greek prefixes

deca- (da):	10
hecto- (h):	100
kilo- (k):	1,000
mega- (M):	1,000,000

Greek prefixes denote multiples.

Prefixes with Standard Measures

Length

The standard measure is the meter (m).

1 kilometer (km)	= 1,000 meters (m)
0.001 kilometer (km)	= 1 meter (m)
1 millimeter (mm)	= 0.001 meter (m)
1,000 millimeters (mm)	= 1 meter (m)
1 centimeter (cm)	= 0.01 meter (m)
100 centimeters (cm)	= 1 meter (m)

Volume

The standard measure is the liter (L).

1 milliliter (ml)	= 0.001 liter (L)
1,000 milliliters (ml)	= 1 liter (L)
1 microliter (mcl)	= 0.000001 liter (L)
1,000,000 microliters (mcl)	= 1 liter (L)
1 deciliter (dl)	= 0.1 liter (L)
10 deciliters (dl)	= 1 liter (L)

Weight

The standard measure is the gram (g).

1 kilogram (kg)	= 1,000 grams (g)
0.001 kilogram (kg)	= 1 gram (g)
1 milligram (mg)	= 0.001 gram (g)
1,000 milligrams (mg)	= 1 gram (g)
1 microgram (mcg)	= 0.000001 gram (g)
1,000,000 micrograms (mcg)	= 1 gram (g)

Apothecary System

The apothecary system was developed after the avoirdupois system to enable fine weighings of medications. Today, the apothecary system is used only for a few medications, such as aspirin, acetaminophen, and phenobarbital.

Weight

The standard measure for weight is the grain (gr).

Pound	Ounces	Drams	Scruples	Grains
1 =	12 =	96 =	288 =	5,760
	1 =	8 =	24 =	480
		1 =	3 =	60
			1 =	20

Volume

The standard measure for volume is the minim (m.).

Gallons	Pints	Fluid ounces	Fluid drams	Minims
1 =	8 =	128 =	1,024 =	61,440
	1 =	16 =	128 =	7,680
		1 =	8 =	480
			1 =	60

Avoirdupois System

This system is mainly used in measuring the bulk medications encountered in manufacturing. The pounds-to-ounces equivalent is different in the apothecary and avoirdupois systems. The avoirdupois system is most commonly used to measure weight, and the apothecary system is most commonly used to measure volume. The technician should take note of the difference in symbols used for the two systems. Another important point to note is that fluid ounces, which measure volume, are often mistakenly shortened to "ounces," which is actually a measure of weight. Because ounces measure weight, the technician must pay close attention to the measure he or she is working with and convert accordingly.

Weight

The standard measure for weight is the grain (gr).

Pound	Ounces	Grains
(lb)	(oz)	(gr)
1 =	16 =	7,000
	1 =	437.5

Household System

The household system is the most commonly used system of measuring liquids in outpatient settings. The measuring equipment usually consists of commonly used home utensils (teaspoons, tablespoons, etc.).

1 teaspoonful (tsp) = 5 ml

1 dessertspoonful = 10 ml

1 tablespoonful (TBS) = 15 ml = 0.5 fluid ounces (fl oz)

1 wineglassful = 60 ml = 2 fl oz

1 teacupful = 120 ml = 4 fl oz

1 glassful/cupful = 240 ml = 8 fl oz

3 tsp = 1 TBS

2 TBS = 1 fl oz

8 fl oz = 1 cup

2 cups = 1 pint (pt)

2 pt = 1 quart (qt)

4 qt = 1 gallon (gal)

The term *drop* is used commonly; however, caution should be used when working with this measure, especially with potent medications. The volume of a drop depends not only on the nature of the liquid but also on the size, shape, and position of the dropper. To accurately measure small amounts of liquid, use a 1 ml syringe (with milliliter markings) instead of a dropper. Eyedrops are an exception to this rule; they are packaged in a manner to deliver a correctly sized droplet.

Equivalencies Between Systems

The systems that have been described lack a close relationship among their units. For this reason, the preferred system of measuring is the metric system. The tables of weights and measures below give the approximate equivalencies used in practice.

Length Measures

1 meter (m)	= 39.37 (39.4) inches (in)
1 inch (in)	= 2.54 centimeters (cm)
1 micron (mc)	= 0.000001 meter (m)

Volume Measures   *1 cup = 240 mL*

1 milliliter (ml)	= 16.23 minims (m.)
1 fluid ounce (fl oz)	= 29.57 (30) milliliters (ml)
1 liter (L)	= 33.8 fluid ounces (fl oz)
1 pint (pt)	= 473.167 (480) milliliters (ml)
1 gallon (cong)	= 3785.332 (3785) milliliters (ml)

Weight Measures

1 kilogram (kg)	= 2.2 pounds (lb)
1 pound (avoir) (lb)	= 453.59 (454) grams (g)
1 ounce (avoir) (oz)	= 28.35 (28) grams (g)
1 ounce (apoth) (oz)	= 31.1 (31) grams (g)
1 gram (g)	= 15.432 (15) grains (gr)
1 grain (gr)	= 65 milligrams (mg)
1 ounce (avoir) (oz)	= 437.5 grains (gr)
1 ounce (apoth)	= 480 grains (gr)

Temperature Conversion

Temperature is measured in the number of degrees centigrade (°C), also known as degrees Celsius, or the number of degrees Fahrenheit (°F). The following equation shows the relationship between degrees centigrade and degrees Fahrenheit:

$$[9(°C)] = [5(°F)] - 160°$$

Example: Convert 110°F to °C.

[9(°C)]	=	[5(110°F)] – 160°
°C	=	(550 – 160)/9
°C	=	43.3°

Example: Convert 15°C to °F

[9(15°C)]	=	[5(°F)] – 160°
(135 + 160)/5	=	°F
59°	=	°F

Conversion Between Systems

The following steps are necessary to find out how many kilograms are in 44 lbs:

1. Write down the statement of equivalency between the two units of measure and make sure that the unit corresponding with the unknown in the question is on the right.

   2.2 lbs = 1 kg

2. Write down the problem with the unknown underneath the equivalency.

   Equivalency: 2.2 lbs = 1 kg

   Problem: 44 lbs = ? kg

3. Cross multiply and divide.

   1 times 44 divided by 2.2 = [(1 × 44)/2.2] = 20 kg

Determining Body Surface Area

The square meter surface area (body surface area) is a measurement that is used instead of kilograms to estimate the amount of medication a patient should receive. Body surface area (BSA) takes into account the patient's weight and height. BSA is always expressed in meters squared (m^2) and is frequently used to dose chemotherapy agents. The following equation is used to determine BSA. When using the equation below, units of weight (W) should be kilograms (kg) and height (H) should be centimeters.

$$BSA = (W^{0.5378}) \times (H^{0.3964}) \times (0.024265)$$

Ratio and Proportion

A ratio states a relationship between two quantities.

Example: 5 g of dextrose in 100 ml of water (this solution is often abbreviated "D5W").

A proportion is two equal ratios.

Example: 5 g of dextrose in 100 ml of a D5W solution equals 50 g of dextrose in 1,000 ml of a D5W solution;

or

$$\frac{5 \text{ g}}{100 \text{ ml}} = \frac{50 \text{ g}}{1000 \text{ ml}}$$

A proportion consists of two unit (or term) types (e.g., kilograms and liters, or milligrams and milliliters). If three of the four terms are known, the fourth term can be calculated.

Problem Solving by the Ratio and Proportion Method

The ratio and proportion method is an accurate and simple way to solve certain problems. To use this method, the technician should learn how to arrange the terms correctly and must know how to multiply and divide.

There is more than one way to write a proportion. The most common is the following:

$$\frac{\text{Term \#1}}{\text{Term \#2}} = \frac{\text{Term \#3}}{\text{Term \#4}}$$

This expression is read, "Term #1 is to Term #2 as Term #3 is to Term #4."

By cross multiplying, the proportion can now be written as follows:

(Term #1) × (Term #4) = (Term #2) × (Term #3)

Example 1: How many grams of dextrose are in 10 ml of a solution containing 50 g of dextrose in 100 ml of water (D50W)?

The following steps are necessary to solve this problem:

1. Determine which is the known ratio and which is the unknown ratio. In this example, the known ratio is "50 g of dextrose in 100 ml of solution." The unknown ratio is "X g of dextrose in 10 ml of solution."

2. Write the unknown ratio (terms #1 and #2) on the left side of the proportion. Be sure that the unknown term is on the top.

$$\frac{X \text{ g}}{10 \text{ ml}} = \frac{\text{Term \#3}}{\text{Term \#4}}$$

3. Write the known ratio (terms #3 and #4) on the right side of the proportion. The units of both ratios must be the same—the units in the numerators and the units in the denominators must match. In this case, that means grams in the numerator and milliliters in the denominator. If units of the numerators or the denominators differ, then a conversion to the same units must be completed.

$$\frac{X \text{ g}}{10 \text{ ml}} = \frac{50 \text{ g}}{100 \text{ ml}}$$

4. Cross multiply.

$$X \text{ g} \times 100 \text{ ml} = 50 \text{ g} \times 10 \text{ ml}$$

5. Divide each side of the equation by the known number on the left side of the equation. This will leave only the unknown value on the left side of the equation:

$$X \text{ g} = \frac{50 \text{ g} \times 10 \text{ ml}}{100 \text{ ml}}$$

6. Simplify the right side of the equation to solve for X grams:

Answer: $X \text{ g} = 5 \text{ g}$

Example 2: The technician needs to prepare a 500-mg chloramphenicol dose in a syringe. The concentration of chloramphenicol solution is 250 mg/ml. How many milliliters should be drawn up into the syringe?

The following steps are necessary to solve this problem:

1. Determine the known and unknown ratios.

Known: $\dfrac{1 \text{ ml}}{250 \text{ mg}}$

Unknown: $\dfrac{X \text{ ml}}{500 \text{ mg}}$

2. Write the proportion:

$$\frac{X \text{ ml}}{500 \text{ mg}} = \frac{1 \text{ ml}}{250 \text{ mg}}$$

3. Cross multiply:

$$X \text{ ml} \times 250 \text{ mg} = 1 \text{ ml} \times 500 \text{ mg}$$

4. Divide:

$$X \text{ ml} = \frac{1 \text{ ml} \times 500 \text{ mg}}{250 \text{ mg}}$$

5. Simplify:

$X \text{ ml} = 2 \text{ ml}$

Answer: Draw up 2 ml in the syringe to prepare a 500-mg dose of chloramphenicol.

Concentration and Dilution

Terminology

■ 5% dextrose in water is the same as D5W

■ 0.9% sodium chloride (NaCl) is the same as normal saline (NS).

■ Half-normal saline is half the strength of normal saline (0.9% NaCl), or 0.45% NaCl. It may also be referred to as 0.5 NS or 1/2 NS.

Concentration Expressed as a Percentage

The concentration of one substance in another may be expressed as a percentage or a ratio strength.

As stated earlier in this chapter, concentrations expressed as percentages are determined using one of the following formulas:

1. Percent weight-in-weight (w/w) is the grams of a drug in 100 grams of the product.

2. Percent weight-in-volume (w/v) is the grams of a drug in 100 ml of the product.

3. Percent volume-in-volume (v/v) is the milliliters of drug in 100 ml of the product.

Example 1:

0.9% sodium chloride (w/v) = 0.9 g of sodium chloride in 100 ml of solution.

Example 2:

5% dextrose in water (w/v) = 5 g of dextrose in 100 ml of solution.

Example 3:

How many grams of dextrose are in 1 L of D5W?

The following steps of the ratio and proportion method are necessary to solve this problem:

Known ratio: D5W means $\dfrac{5 \text{ g}}{100 \text{ ml}}$

Unknown ratio: $\dfrac{X \text{ g}}{1 \text{ L}}$

1. Write the proportion:

$$\frac{X \text{ g}}{1 \text{ L}} = \frac{5 \text{ g}}{100 \text{ ml}}$$

2. It is not time yet to cross multiply. First, convert the denominator of either term so both are the same. Because we know that 1 L = 1,000 ml, the

unlike terms should be converted as follows:

$$\frac{X\,g}{1000\ ml} = \frac{5\,g}{100\ ml}$$

3. Now that the units are both in the same order and the units across from each other are the same, cross multiply:

$$X\,g \times 100\ ml = 5\ g \times 1000\ ml$$

4. Divide:

$$X\,g = \frac{5\,g \times 1000\ ml}{100\ ml}$$

5. Simplify:

$$X\,g = 50\ g$$

There are 50 g of dextrose in 1 L of D5W.

Here are a few suggestions for solving concentration and dilution problems.

1. Calculate the number of grams in 100 ml of solution first. That is the "known" side of the ratio.
2. Calculate the number of grams in the volume requested in the problem by setting up a ratio.
3. Check to make sure the units are in the same order in the ratio.
4. Make sure the units that are across from each other in the ratio are the same.
5. After arriving at the answer, convert it to the requested units.

Concentration Expressed as a Ratio Strength

Concentrations of weak solutions are frequently expressed as ratio strength.

Example: Epinephrine is available in three concentrations: 1:1,000 (read "one to one thousand"); 1:10,000; and 1:200.

A concentration of 1:1,000 means there is 1 g of epinephrine in 1,000 ml of solution.

What does a 1:200 concentration of epinephrine mean?

It means 1 g of epinephrine in 200 ml of solution.

What does a 1:10,000 concentration of epinephrine mean?

It means 1 g of epinephrine in 10,000 ml of solution.

The pharmacy technician can use this definition of ratio strength to set up the ratios needed to solve problems.

Dilutions Made from Stock Solutions

Stock solutions are concentrated solutions used to prepare various dilutions of the original stock solution. To prepare a solution of a desired concentration, the technician must calculate the quantity of stock solution that must be mixed with diluent to prepare the final product.

Calculating Dilutions

Example 1: A 10% NaCl stock solution is available. The technician needs to prepare 200 ml of a 0.5% NaCl solution. How many milliliters of the stock solution does the technician need to make this preparation? How much more water does the technician need to add to produce the final product?

The following steps are necessary to solve this problem:

1. Calculate how many grams of NaCl are in the requested final product.

$$\frac{X\ g\ NaCl}{200\ ml\ soln} = \frac{0.5\ g\ NaCl}{100\ ml\ soln}$$

Therefore, 200 ml of 0.5% NaCl solution contains 1 g of NaCl.

2. Calculate how many milliliters of the stock solution will contain the amount calculated in step 1 (i.e., 1 g):

Remember, 10% means the solution contains 10 g/100 ml.

$$\frac{X\ ml}{1\ g} = \frac{100\ ml}{10\ g}$$
$$X\ ml = 10\ ml$$

The first part of the answer is 10 ml of stock solution.

3. Calculate how much water is needed to finish preparing the solution.

Keep in mind the following formula:

(final volume) – (stock solution volume) = (volume of water)

Therefore, for the problem "200 ml – 10 ml = 190 ml of water," the second part of the answer is 190 ml of water.

Example 2: The technician has to prepare 500 ml of a 0.45% NaCl solution from a 10% NaCl stock solution. How much stock solution and water are needed?

The following steps are necessary to solve this problem:

1. Calculate how many grams of NaCl are in the requested volume. In other words, 500 ml of a 0.45% NaCl solution contains how much NaCl?

$$\frac{X \text{ g NaCl}}{500 \text{ ml}} = \frac{0.45 \text{ g}}{100 \text{ ml}}$$

$$X \text{ g} \times 100 \text{ ml} = 0.45 \text{ g} \times 500 \text{ ml}$$

$$X \text{ g} = \frac{0.45 \text{ g} \times 500 \text{ ml}}{100 \text{ ml}}$$

$$X \text{ g} = 2.25 \text{ g}$$

2. Calculate how many milliliters of stock solution will contain the amount in step 1 (i.e., 2.25 g)?

$$\frac{X \text{ ml}}{2.25 \text{ g}} = \frac{100 \text{ ml}}{10 \text{ g}}$$

$$X \text{ ml} \times 10 \text{ g} = 2.25 \text{ g} \times 100 \text{ ml}$$

$$X \text{ ml} = \frac{2.25 \text{ g} \times 100 \text{ ml}}{10 \text{ g}}$$

$$X \text{ ml} = 22.5 \text{ ml}$$

The technician will need 22.5 ml of stock solution.

3. Calculate how much water the technician will need.

(Final volume) − (stock solution volume) = volume of water

500 ml − 22.5 ml = 477.5 ml water

Answer: The technician will need 22.5 ml of stock solution and 477.5 ml of water to make the final product.

Dosage and Flow Rate Calculations

Dosage Calculations

Basic Principles

1. The technician should always look for what is being asked:
   - Number of doses
   - Total amount of drug
   - Size of a dose

   Given any two of the above, the technician can solve for the third.

2. Number of doses, total amount of drug, and size of dose are related in the following way:

$$\text{Number of doses} = \frac{\text{Total amount of drug}}{\text{Size of dose}}$$

This proportion can also be rearranged as follows:

Total amount of drug = (number of doses) × (size of dose)

or

$$\text{Size of dose} = \frac{\text{Total amount of drug}}{\text{Number of doses}}$$

Dosage calculations can be based on weight, BSA, or age.

Calculating Dose Based on Weight

Dose (in mg) = [dose per unit of weight (in mg/kg)] × [Weight of patient (in kg)]

Dose/day (in mg/day) = [dose/kg per day (in mg/kg per day)] × [Weight of patient (in kg)]

To find the size of each dose, the technician should divide the total dose per day by the number of doses per day, as illustrated in the following formula:

$$\text{Size of Dose} = \frac{\text{Total amount of drug}}{\text{Number of doses}}$$

Calculating Dose Based on BSA

As noted previously in this chapter, BSA is expressed as meters squared (m^2). To calculate the amount of a dose on the basis of BSA, the technician should simply multiply the BSA in m^2 times the dose per m^2 as provided in the order or other labeling.

Calculating Dose Based on Age

The following is an example of information that might be found on the label of an over-the-counter children's medication:

St. Joseph's Cough Syrup for Children

Pediatric Antitussive Syrup

Active ingredient: Dextromethorphan hydrobromide 7.5 mg per 5 ml

Indications: For relief of coughing associated with colds and flu for up to 8 hours

Actions: Antitussive

Warnings: Should not be administered to children for persistent or chronic cough, such as occurs with asthma or emphysema, or when cough is accompanied by excessive secretions (except under physician's advice)

How supplied: Cherry-flavored syrup in plastic bottles of 2 and 4 fl oz

Dosage: (see table below)

Age	Weight	Dosage
Under 2 yr	below 27 lb	As directed by physician
2 to under 6 yr	27 to 45 lb	1 tsp every 6 to 8 h (not to exceed 4 tsp daily)

| 6 to under 12 yr | 46 to 83 lb | 2 tsp every 6 to 8 h (not to exceed 8 tsp daily) |
| 12 yr and older | 84 lb and greater | 4 tsp every 6 to 8 h (not to exceed 16 tsp daily) |

To determine the dose, the technician should compare the child's age to the instructions provided on the drug label.

IV Flow Rate Calculations

Using flow rates, the technician can calculate the volume of fluid or the amount of drug a patient will be receiving over a certain period. Prefilled IV bags are available in the following volumes: 25, 50, 100, 250, 500, and 1,000 ml.

Calculating Volume of Fluid

Daily volume of fluid (in ml/day) = [Flow rate (in ml/h)] × [24 h/day]

Calculation of IV Flow (Drip) Rates

Calculation of IV flow (drip) rates is necessary to ensure that patients are getting the amount of medication the physician ordered. For example, if an order is written as "25,000 units of heparin in 250 ml D5W to infuse at 1,000 units/h," what is the correct rate of infusion (in ml/h)?

$$\text{Concentration of IV} = \frac{\text{Total amount of drug}}{\text{Total volume}}$$

$$\text{Concentration of IV} = \frac{25,000 \text{ units heparin}}{250 \text{ ml D5W}}$$

$$\text{Concentration of IV} = 100 \text{ units/ml of D5W}$$

Once the technician has calculated the concentration per milliliter, he or she can determine exactly what the rate should be by using the following formula:

$$\text{IV Rate} = \frac{\text{Dose desired}}{\text{Concentration of IV}}$$

$$\text{IV Rate} = \frac{(1,000 \text{ units/h})}{(100 \text{ units/ml})}$$

$$\text{IV Rate} = 10 \text{ ml/h}$$

Statistics

The arithmetic mean is a value that is calculated by dividing the sum of a set of numbers by the total number of number sets. This value is also referred to as an *average*. The following formula is used to determine the average:

$$M = \frac{\sum X}{N}$$

Σ = sum

M = mean (average)

X = one value in set of data

N = number of values X in data set

Using the formula, the following steps help one to calculate the arithmetic mean age of five pharmacists whose ages are 25, 28, 33, 47, and 54 years.

1. Calculate the sum of all ages.
2. Divide the sum by total number of pharmacists

$$\frac{25 + 28 + 33 + 47 + 54}{5} = \frac{187}{5} = 37.4 \text{ years}$$

The *median* is a value in an ordered set of values below and above which there are an equal number of values. When an even number of measurements are arranged according to size, the median is defined as the mean of the values of the two measurements that are nearest to the middle. In the previous example, the median age is 33 years.

Ideal Body Weight

IBW is required to determine the estimated creatinine clearance of an individual patient. The estimated creatinine clearance is needed to determine the appropriate dose of renally excreted medications, such as tobramycin. The formula for calculating the IBW for a male is the following:

$$\text{IBW male (kg)} = 50 + \frac{(2.3 \times \text{height in inches})}{5 \text{ feet}}$$

The formula for calculating the IBW for a female is the following:

$$\text{IBW female (kg)} = 45.5 + \frac{(2.3 \times \text{height in inches})}{5 \text{ feet}}$$

Practice Calculations 1

1. Convert IV to its Arabic equivalent: 4
2. Convert III to its Arabic equivalent: 3
3. Write 4/5 as a decimal fraction: 0.8
4. Write the fraction form of 0.4: 4/10 = 2/5
5. Express 75% as a fraction: 3/4
6. Write 0.42 as a percentage: 42%
7. Express 1/2 as a percentage: 50%
8. Write the fraction form of 0.2: 2/10 = 1/5
9. Express XXII in Arabic numbers: 22

10. Express 1 1/4 in decimal form: 1.25

11. The standard metric system measure for weight is the gram

12. The standard metric system measure for length is the meter

13. The standard metric system measure for volume is the liter

14. 1 m = 0.001 km

15. 1 ml = 0.001 L

16. 1 g = 0.001 kg

17. 1 mg = 0.001 g

18. 1 mg = 1000 mcg

19. 1 mg = 1,000 mg

20. 1 L = 1000 ml

21. 1 TBS = 3 tsp

22. 1 fl oz = 30 ml

23. 1 TBS = 15 ml

24. 15 ml = 3 tsp

25. 1/2 cup = 4 fl oz

26. 100 ml = 0.1 L

27. 2 kg = 4.4 lb

28. 1 pt = ½ qt

29. 1 qt = 4 cups

30. 1 kg = 1000 g

31. 1 tsp = 5 ml

32. 5 gr = 325 mg

33. 4 cups = 960 ml

34. 85 kg = 187 lb

35. 60 ml = 2 fl oz

36. 50 mg = 0.77 gr

37. 25 mg = 0.25 g

38. 2 TBS = 6 tsp

39. 1 fl oz = 4 TBS

40. 4 qt = 8 pt

41. 100 ml = 0.42 cups

42. 20 ml = 4 tsp

43. 40 ml = 2.67 TBS

44. 150 mg = 0.15 g

45. 3 gal = 12 qt

46. 2.5 pt = 1182.5 ml

47. 30 kg = 66 lb

48. 725 mg = 0.725 g

49. 10 ml = 2 tsp

50. 9 tsp = 3 TBS

Practice Calculations 2

1. 4% (w/w) = 4g / 100 g

   12% (w/v) = 12 g / 100 mL

   0.75% (v/v) = .75 ml / 100 ml

2. A patient needs a 350-mg dose of amikacin. How many milliliters does the technician need to draw from a vial containing 100 mg/2 ml of amikacin? *7*

3. A suspension of naladixic acid contains 250 mg/5 ml. The syringe contains 20 ml. What is the dose (in milligrams) contained in the syringe? *1000*

4. How many milligrams of neomycin are in 250 ml of a 1% neomycin solution? *2500*

5. 1/2 NS = 0.45 g NaCl / 100 ml solution

6. How many grams of pumpkin are in 200 ml of a 25% pumpkin juice suspension? *50*

7. Express 2.5% hydrocortisone cream as a ratio. (Remember that solids, such as creams, are usually expressed as w/w.) *2.5 g/100g*

8. The technician has a solution labeled "D10W/NS."

   a) How many grams of NaCl are in 100 ml of this solution? *0.9 g*

   b) How many milliliters of this solution contain 10 g dextrose? *100 mL*

9. A syringe is labeled "inamrinone 5 mg/ml, 10 ml." How many milligrams of inamrinone are in the syringe? *50*

10. Boric acid 5:100 is written on a prescription. This is the same as 5 g boric acid in 100 mL solution.

11. How much epinephrine is necessary to prepare 20 ml of a 1:1000 epinephrine solution? *0.02 g*

12. Calculate the amounts of boric acid and zinc sulfate to fill the following prescription:

    R   *0.1 g   10 g*
    Zinc sulfate 0.1%
    Boric acid   1:10
    Distilled water qs. ad 100 ml

13. Use the following concentrations to solve the problems:

    Gentamicin 80 mg/ml
    Magnesium sulfate   50%
    Atropine   1:200

a) 160 mg gentamicin = __2__ ml

b) 10 mg atropine = __2__ ml

c) __60__ g magnesium sulfate = 120 ml

Practice Calculations 3

1. The technician needs to prepare 2 L of 0.25% acetic acid irrigation solution. The stock concentration of acetic acid is 25%.

    a. How many milliliters of stock solution are needed?   20

    b. How many milliliters of sterile water have to be added?   1980

2. A drug order requires 50 ml of a 2% neomycin solution.

    a. How much neomycin concentrate (1 g/2 ml) is needed to fill the order?   2

    b. How many milliliters of sterile water need to be added to the concentrate before dispensing the drug?   48

3. a. Calculate the amount of atropine stock solution (concentration 0.5%) needed to compound the following prescription: 60

    R

    Atropine sulfate   1:1000

    Sterile water qs ad   300 ml

    b. How much sterile water has to be added to complete the order?   240

4. How many tablets have to be dispensed for the following prescription?

    R

    Obecalp ii tablets tid for 14 days   84

5. How many 2-tsp doses can a patient take from a bottle containing 4 fl oz?   12

6. A patient is receiving a total daily dose of 1 g of acyclovir. How many milligrams of acyclovir is he receiving per dose if he takes the drug five times a day?   200

7. The recommended dose of erythromycin to treat an ear infection is 50 mg/kg per day given q6h. Answer the following questions regarding this drug:

    a. If a child weighs 15 kg, how much erythromycin should he receive per day?   750

    b. How much drug will he receive per dose?   187.5

8. The dose of prednisone for replacement therapy is 2 mg/m^2 per dose. The drug is administered twice daily. What is the daily prednisone dose for a 1.2-m^2 person?   4.8

9. An aminophylline drip is running at 1 mg/kg per hour in a 12-kg child. How much aminophylline is the child receiving per day?   288

10. A child with an opiate overdose needs naloxone. The recommended starting dose is 5–10 mcg/kg. The doctor writes for "0.3 mg naloxone stat." Answer the following questions on the basis of the child's weight of 35 kg:

    a. What is the dosage range of the starting dose?   175·350

    b. On the basis of the answer to "a," does 0.3 mg sound like a reasonable dose?   yes

11. An IV fluid containing NS is running at 125 ml/h.

    a. How much fluid is the patient receiving per day?   3,000

    b. How many 1 L bags will be needed per day?   3

12. A patient has two IVs running: an aminophylline drip at 22 ml/h and saline at 40 ml/h. How much fluid is the patient receiving per day from his IVs?   1488

13. a. You prepare a solution by adding 1 g of Bronkospaz to 1 L of NS. What is the concentration of Bronkospaz?   1,000 ml / 1,000 g

    b. If the solution of Bronkospaz you made in "a" runs at 40 ml/h, how much Bronkospaz is the patient receiving per day?   960

    c. If a 50-kg patient should receive 1 mg/kg per hour, will the dose in "b" be appropriate?   NO

Answers to Practice Calculations 1

1. 4
2. 3
3. 0.8
4. 2/5
5. 3/4
6. 42%
7. 50%
8. 1/5
9. 22
10. 1.25
11. gram
12. meter

13.	liter
14.	0.001
15.	0.001
16.	0.001
17.	0.001
18.	1000
19.	1,000
20.	1,000
21.	3
22.	29.57 (30)
23.	15
24.	3
25.	4
26.	0.1
27.	4.4
28.	1/2
29.	4
30.	1,000
31.	5
32.	325
~~33.~~	946 960
34.	187
35.	2
36.	0.77
37.	0.025
38.	6
39.	6
40.	8
41.	0.42
42.	4
43.	2.67
44.	0.15
45.	12
46.	1,182.5
47.	66
48.	0.725
49.	2
50.	3

Answers to Practice Calculations 2

1. 4 g/100 g
   12 g/100 ml
   0.75 ml/100 ml
2. 7 ml
3. 1,000 mg
4. 2,500 mg
5. 0.45 g/100 ml
6. 50 g
7. 2.5 g/100 g
8. a. 0.9 g
   b. 100 ml
9. 50 mg
10. 5 g in 100 ml
11. 0.02 g or 20 mg
12. 0.1 g zinc sulfate and 10 g boric acid
13. a. 2 ml
    b. 2 ml
    c. 60 g

Answers to Practice Calculations 3

1. a. 20 ml stock solution
   b. 1,980 ml sterile water
2. a. 2 ml stock solution
   b. 48 ml stock solution
3. a. 60 ml stock solution
   b. 240 ml sterile water
4. 84 tablets
5. 12 doses
6. 200 mg per dose
7. a. 750 mg per day
   b. 187.5 mg per dose
8. 4.8 mg per day
9. 288 mg per day
10. a. Acceptable dosage range: 175–350 mcg
    b. Yes, it falls within the accepted calculated range.
11. a. 3,000 ml per day
    b. Three 1 L bags per day
12. 1,488 ml per day

13.   a. 1,000 mg/1,000 ml or 1 mg/ml or
        1 g/1,000 ml or 1 g/L or 1:1,000

        b. 960 mg/day

        c. No, the dose is lower than would be
        expected (1,200 mg/day).

Suggested Reading

From *Manual for Pharmacy Technicians,* 3rd ed.:

Pharmacy Calculations: See Chapter 5—Pharmacy
Calculations.

Commonly Prescribed Medications

Respiratory System

TABLE 1: AGENTS USED TO TREAT ASTHMA AND CHRONIC OBSTRUCTIVE PULMONARY DISEASE		
Generic Name	**Brand Name**	**Common Side Effects**
Short-acting bronchodilators		
Albuterol	Proventil, Ventolin,	Tremors, nervousness, fast heart rate
	Proventil HFA,	"
	Ventolin HFA, Volmax	"
Metaproterenol	Alupent	"
Pirbuterol	Maxair	"
Levalbuterol	Xopenex	"
Long-acting bronchodilators		
Salmeterol	Serevent	Tremors, nervousness, fast heart rate
Formeterol	Foradil	"
Theophylline	various brands	Nausea, vomiting, fast heart rate, headache, insomnia
Inhaled corticosteroids		
Triamcinolone	Azmacort	Thrush, hoarseness
Budesonide	Pulmicort	"
Fluticasone	Flovent	"
Flunisolide	Aerobid, Aerobid-M	"
Beclomethasone	Beclovent, Vanceril, Q-Var	"
Mast cell stabilizers		
Nedocromil	Tilade	Dizziness, headache, rash
Cromolyn sodium	Intal	"
Anticholinergics		
Ipratropium	Atrovent	Flushing, dry mouth, constipation, confusion
Leukotriene inhibitors		
Zafirlukast	Accolate	Headache, cough, abdominal pain
Montelukast	Singulair	"

Generic Name	Brand Name	Common Side Effects
Zileuton	Zyflo	Headache, cough, abdominal pain

Combination agents

Salmeterol/Fluticasone	Advair	
Ipratropium/Albuterol	Combivent	

TABLE 2: ANTIHISTAMINES

Generic Name	Brand Name	Availability
First-generation antihistamines		
Chlorpheniramine	Chlor-Trimeton	OTC
Clemastine	Tavist, Tavist-1	OTC
Diphenhydramine	Benadryl	OTC
Hydroxyzine	Atarax	Rx
Promethazine	Phenergan	Rx
Second-generation antihistamines		
Cetirizine	Zyrtec	Rx
Loratadine	Claritin	OTC
Third-generation antihistamines		
Desloratadine	Clarinex	Rx
Fexofenadine	Allegra	Rx

Note: OTC = over the counter; Rx = by prescription.

TABLE 3: MISCELLANEOUS RESPIRATORY MEDICATIONS

Generic Name	Brand Name	Indication
Dextromethorphan	Various OTC	Antitussive
Guaifenesin	Various OTC	Expectorant

Central Nervous System

TABLE 4: ANTIDEPRESSANTS

Generic Name	Brand Name	Common Side Effects
Tricyclic antidepressants		
Amitriptyline	Elavil	Sedation, dry mouth, blurred vision, constipation, difficulty urinating, dizziness upon standing
Nortriptyline	Pamelor	
Protriptyline	Vivactil	
Imipramine	Tofranil, Tofranil-PM	"

Generic Name	Brand Name	Common Side Effects
Tricyclic antidepressants (cont'd)		
Desipramine	Norpramin	"
Doxepin	Sinequan	"
Clomipramine	Anafranil	"
Monoamine oxidase inhibitors (MAOIs)		
Isocarboxazid	Marplan	Postural hypotension or hypertensive crisis
Phenelzine	Nardil	
Tranylcypromine	Parnate	"
Selective serotonin reuptake inhibitors (SSRIs)		
Fluoxetine	Prozac	Nausea, diarrhea, anorexia
Paroxetine	Paxil	
Sertraline	Zoloft	"
Citalopram	Celexa	"
Escitalopram	Lexapro	"
Fluvoxamine	Luvox	"
Miscellaneous agents		
Nefazodone	Serzone	Same as tricyclics
Trazodone	Desyrel	"
Venlafaxine	Effexor, Effexor-XR	"
Bupropion	Wellbutrin, Wellbutrin-SR, Zyban	Seizures " "
Mirtazapine	Remeron	Agranulocytosis

TABLE 5: ANTIPSYCHOTICS

Generic Name	Brand Name	Dosage Forms
Conventional antipsychotics		
Low-potency		
Chlorpromazine	Thorazine	Tablets, concentrated liquid, suppositories, injection
Thioridazine	Mellaril	Tablets, suspension
Intermediate-potency		
Perphenazine	Trilafon	Tablets, concentrated liquid
Loxapine	Loxitane	Capsules, concentrated liquid
High-potency		
Trifluoperazine	Stelazine	Tablets, concentrated liquid

Generic Name	Brand Name	Dosage Forms
Fluphenazine	Prolixin	Tablets, deconoate injection, liquid, elixir
Thiothixene	Navane	Capsules
Halperidol	Haldol	Tablets, concentrated liquid, injection, deconoate injection

Atypical antipsychotics

Generic Name	Brand Name	Dosage Forms
Clozapine	Clozaril	Tablets
Olanzepine	Zyprexa	Tablets
Risperidone	Riserdal	Tablets, solution
Quetiapine	Seroquel	Tablets
Ziprasidone	Geodon	Capsules
Aripiprazole	Abilify	Tablets

TABLE 6: SEDATIVES AND HYPNOTICS

Generic Name	Brand Name	Uses

Benzodiazepines

Generic Name	Brand Name	Uses
Alprazolam	Xanax	Used for anxiety, sedation
Chlordiazepoxide	Librium	Used for anxiety
Clorazepate	Tranxene	Used for anxiety, sedation
Diazepam	Valium	Used for anxiety, status epilepticus, as muscle relaxant
Lorazepam	Ativan	Used for anxiety, status epilepticus, as muscle relaxant
Midazolam	Versed	Used for sedation in surgical procedures
Oxazepam	Serax	Used for anxiety
Estazolam	Prosom	Used for sedation
Flurazepam	Dalmane	Used for sedation; longest-acting hypnotic
Temazepam	Restoril	Used for sedation
Triazolam	Halcion	Used for sedation; shortest-acting hypnotic
Quazepam	Doral	Used for sedation

Other agents (nonbenzodiazepines)

Generic Name	Brand Name	Uses
Buspirone	Buspar	Low abuse potential, less sedating than benzodiazepine, used for anxiety

Generic Name	Brand Name	Uses
Zolpidem	Ambien	Used for sedation
Zaleplon	Sonata	Used for sedation
Phenobarbital	Luminal	Used for sedation, anticonvulsant
Secobarbital	Seconal	Used for sedation
Chloral hydrate	Aquachloral	Used for procedure sedation

TABLE 7: ANTICONVULSANTS

Generic Name	Trade Name	Seizure Indication
Phenytoin	Dilantin	Status epilepticus, tonic-clonic
Fosphenytoin	Cerebyx	Status epilepticus, tonic-clonic
Ethotoin	Peganone	Status epilepticus, tonic-clonic
Diazepam	Valium	Status epilepticus
Lorazepam	Ativan	Status epilepticus
Clonazepam	Klonopin	Absence, myoclonic
Valproic acid	Depakene	Absence
Divalproex Na	Depakote	Absence, partial
Ethosuximide	Zarontin	Absence
Carbamazepine	Tegretol, Tegretol-XR	Tonic-clonic, partial
Primidone	Mysoline	Tonic-clonic
Gabapentin	Neurontin	Tonic-clonic, partial
Oxcarbazepine	Trileptal	Partial
Lamotrigine	Lamictal	Partial
Felbamate	Felbatol	Partial
Levetiracetam	Keppra	Adjunctive to partial
Tiagabine	Gabitril	Adjunctive to partial
Zonisamide	Zonegran	Adjunctive to partial
Topiramate	Topamax	Adjunctive to tonic-clonic, partial

TABLE 8: ANTI-PARKINSON'S DRUGS

Generic Name	Brand Name	Drug Action
Levodopa/Carbidopa	Sinemet	Increased dopamine in the brain
Tolcapone	Tasmar	Decreased breakdown of levodopa
Entacapone	Comtan	Decreased breakdown of levodopa
Amantadine	Symmetrel	Mimic or increase the activity of dopamine

Generic Name	Brand Name	Drug Action
Bromocriptine	Parlodel	Mimic or increase the activity of dopamine
Pergolide	Permax	Mimic or increase the activity of dopamine
Selegiline	Eldepryl	Mimic or increase the activity of dopamine
Benztropine	Cogentin	Anticholinergic effects
Biperiden	Akineton	Anticholinergic effects
Procyclidine	Kemadrin	Anticholinergic effects
Trihexyphenidyl	Artane	Anticholinergic effects

Cardiovascular System

TABLE 9: ANTIHYPERLIPIDEMICS

Generic Name	Trade Name	Common Side Effects
Bile acid sequestrants		
Cholestyramine	Questran	Constipation, nausea, gas, abdominal cramping
Colestipol	Colestid	
Colesevelam	Welchol	"
HMG-CoA reductase inhibitors (statins)		
Fluvastatin	Lescol	Headache, GI upset, muscle and joint pain, abnormal liver function tests
Lovastatin	Mevacor	
Atorvastatin	Lipitor	
Pravastatin	Pravachol	"
Simvastatin	Zocor	"
Rosuvastatin	Crestor	"
Fibrates		
Gemfibrozil	Lopid	GI symptoms, dizziness, taste disturbances
Fenofibrate	Tricor	
Miscellaneous agents		
Nicotinic acid	Niacin, Niaspan	Flushing, GI symptoms
Niacin/Lovastatin	Advicor	"
Ezetimibe	Zetia	GI symptoms, arthralgia

Note: GI = gastrointestinal.

TABLE 10: MISCELLANEOUS ANTIHYPERTENSIVES

Generic Name	Trade Name	Drug Action
Doxazocin	Cardura	Alpha-1 blocker
Prazocin	Minipress	Alpha-1 blocker
Terazosin	Hytrin	Alpha-1 blocker
Clonidine	Catapres	Alpha-2 agonist
Guanabenz	Wytensin	Alpha-2 agonist
Methyldopa	Aldomet	Alpha-2 agonist
Hydralazine	Apresoline	Direct vasodilator
Minoxidil	Loniten	Direct vasodilator
Reserpine	Serpalan	Peripherally acting adrenergic

TABLE 11: DIURETICS

Generic name	Brand Name	Comments
Thiazide diuretics		
Hydrochlorothiazide (HCTZ)	Hydrodiuril, Microzide	May cause loss of potassium, may alter blood glucose levels
Chlorothiazide	Diuril	
Indapamide	Lozol	"
Chlorthalidone	Hygroton	"
Metolazone	Zaroxolyn	"
Loop diuretics		
Furosemide	Lasix	More potent than thiazides, causes loss of potassium
Bumetanide	Bumex	
Torsemide	Demadex	
Ethacrynic acid	Edecrin	"
Potassium-sparing diuretics		
Spironolactone	Aldactone	Potassium supplements usually not needed. Often used in combination with thiazides to increase potency
Triamterene	Dyrenium	
Combination agents		
Triamterene/HCTZ	Dyazide, Maxzide	Diuretics
Spironolactone/HCTZ	Aldactazide	Diuretics
Amiloride/HCTZ	Moduretic	Diuretics
Losartan/HCTZ	Hyzaar	ARB/diuretic
Lisinopril/HCTZ	Zestoretic	ACE-I/diuretic
Bisoprolol/HCTZ	Zebeta	Beta-blocker/diuretic
Valsartan/HCTZ	Diovan HCT	ARB/diuretic

Note: ARB = angiotesin II receptor blocker; ACE-I = angiotensin-converting enzyme inhibitor.

TABLE 12: BETA-BLOCKERS, ACE INHIBITORS, AND ARBS

Generic Name	Brand Name	Comments
Beta-blockers		
Atenolol	Tenormin	Note - *olol* ending Contraindicated in patients with asthma or diabetes
Metoprolol	Lopressor, Toprol-XL	
Nadolol	Corgard	
Propranolol	Inderal, Inderal LA	
Timolol	Blocadren, Timoptic	"
Carteolol	Cartrol	"
Bisoprolol	Zebeta	"
Pindolol	Visken	"
Sotalol	Betapace	"
Acebutolol	Sectral	"
Carvedilol	Coreg	"
Labetolol	Normodyne, Trandate	"
ACE inhibitors (ACE-Is)		
Captopril	Capoten	Note - *pril* ending May cause dry cough, may not require potassium supplements.
Benazepril	Lotensin	
Enalapril	Vasotec	
Fosinopril	Monopril	
Lisinopril	Prinivil, Zestril	Patients with diabetes may use for kidney protective qualities
Quinapril	Accupril	
Ramipril	Altace	
Tramdolapril	Mavik	"
Perindopril	Aceon	"
Moexipril	Univasc	"
Angiotensin II receptor blockers (ARBs)		
Losartan	Cozaar	Note - *artan* ending Does not cause dry cough Effects similar to ACE-Is
Valsartan	Diovan	
Irbesartan	Avapro	
Candesartan	Atacand	"
Telmisartan	Micardis	"
Eprosartan	Teveten	"
Olmesartan	Benicar	"

TABLE 13: CALCIUM CHANNEL BLOCKERS

Generic Name	Brand Name	Comments
Dihydropyridines		
Amlodipine	Norvasc	Note –*dipine* ending Headache, flushing, and gum overgrowth are side effects
Nifedipine	Procardia XL, Adalat CC	
Felodipine	Plendil	"
Isradipine	DynaCirc	"
Nicardipine	Cardene SR	"
Nisoldipine	Sular	"
Nimodipine	Nimotop	"
Nondihydropyridines		
Diltiazem	Cardizem (SR, CD), Tiazac, Dilacor XR	Nausea, headache are common
Verapamil	Calan SR, Verelan, Isoptin SR, Covera HS	"

TABLE 14: ANTIARRHYTHMICS

Generic Name	Trade Name	Class
Lidocaine	Xylocaine	Class I, Group IB
Tocainide	Tonocard	Class I, Group IB
Mexilitine	Mexitil	Class I, Group IB
Quinidine	Quinaglute, Quinidex	Class I, Group IA
Procainamide	Procan	Class I, Group IA
Disopyramide	Norpace	Class I, Group IA
Flecainide	Tambocor	Class I, Group IC
Bretylium		Class III
Amiodarone	Cordarone, Pacerone	Class III
Sotalol	Betapace	Class III

TABLE 15: MISCELLANEOUS CARDIAC DRUGS

Generic Name	Trade Name	Indication
Nitroglycerin	Various	Angina
Isosorbide dinitrate	Dilatrate, Isordil, Sorbitrate	Angina
Isosorbide mononitrate	Imdur, Ismo, Monoket	Angina
Digoxin	Lanoxin	Heart failure

TABLE 16: ANTICOAGULANTS

Generic Name	Trade Name	Class
Warfarin	Coumadin	Coumarin
Heparin		Unfractionated heparin
Enoxaparin	Lovenox	Low molecular weight heparin
Dalteparin	Fragmin	Low molecular weight heparin
Tinzaparin	Innohep	Low molecular weight heparin

Gastrointestinal System

TABLE 17: DRUGS USED TO TREAT GASTRO-ESOPHAGEAL REFLUX DISEASE

Proton pump inhibitors

Generic Name	Brand Name	Dosage Forms
Omeprazole	Prilosec	Capsule
Pantoprazole	Protonix	Tablet, injection
Lansoprazole	Prevacid	Capsule, suspension
Rabeprazole	Aciphex	Tablet
Esomeprazole	Nexium	Capsule

Histamine-2 antagonists

Generic Name	Brand Name	Dosage Forms
Cimetidine	Tagamet	Tablet, oral liquid, injection
Ranitidine	Zantac	Capsule, effervescent granules, syrup, tablet, injection
Famotidine	Pepcid	Capsule, tablet, powder for oral suspension, injection
Nizatidine	Axid	Capsule, tablet

Gastrointestinal stimulants

Generic Name	Brand Name	Dosage Forms
Metoclopramide	Reglan	Tablet, oral solution, syrup, injection

Musculoskeletal System

TABLE 18: NONSTEROIDAL ANTI-INFLAMMATORY AGENTS

Generic Name	Brand Name	Comments
Ibuprofen	Motrin, Advil	Note -profen ending
Ketoprofen	Orudis, Oruvail	"
Flurbiprofen	Ansaid	"
Diclofenac	Voltaren	
Sulindac	Clinoril	
Etodolac	Lodine	
Ketorolac	Toradol	Indicated for short-term use only
Naproxen	Naprosyn, Naprelan	
Mecloxicam	Mobic	
Piroxicam	Feldene	
Oxaprozin	Daypro	
Indomethacin	Indocin	Used to treat gout
Nabumetone	Relafen	

Generic Name	Brand Name	Comments

Cox-2 inhibitors

Celecoxib	Celebrex	Note -coxib ending
Rofecoxib	Vioxx	"
Valdecoxib	Bextra	"

TABLE 19: ANALGESICS

Generic Name	Trade Name	Dosage Forms
Major opiates		
Morphine	Various	Tablet, sustained-release tablet, injection, oral solution, suppository
Hydromorphone	Dilaudid	Tablet, oral liquid, injection, suppository
Meperidine	Demerol	Tablet, syrup, injection
Fentanyl	Sublimaze, Duragesic, Actiq, Fentanyl Oralet	Injection, transdermal patch, lozenge
Minor opiates		
Codeine		Tablet, oral solution, injection
Oxycodone	Percolone, Oxycontin, Roxicodone	Tablet, capsule, sustained-release tablet, oral liquid
Propoxyphene	Darvon	Capsule, tablet
Nalbuphine	Nubain	Injection
Butorphanol	Stadol	Injection, nasal spray
Dezocine	Dalgan	Injection
Tramadol	Ultram	Tablet
Non-opiates		
Acetaminophen	Tylenol	Caplet, capsule, tablet, chewable tablet, drops, elixir, oral liquid, suppository, suspension, suspension drops

TABLE 20: NEUROMUSCULAR BLOCKING AGENTS

Generic Name	Trade Name
Succinylcholine	Anectine, Quelicin
Tubocurarine	
Mivacurium	Mivacron
Rocuronium	Zemuron
Pancuronium	Pavulon

Generic Name	Trade Name
Atracurium	Tracrium
Vecuronium	Norcuron
Doxacurium	Nuromax

TABLE 21: SKELETAL MUSCLE RELAXANTS

Generic Name	Trade Name	Dosage Forms
Carisoprodol	Soma	Tablet
Chlorzoxazone	Parafon Forte	Caplet, tablet
Cyclobenzaprine	Flexeril	Tablet
Metaxolone	Skelaxin	Tablet
Methocarbamol	Robaxin	Tablet, injection
Orphenadrine	Norflex	Tablet, sustained-release tablet, injection

Endocrine System

TABLE 22: INSULIN

Insulin Type	Onset of Action	Duration of Action
Rapid-acting		
Lispro	5–15 min.	3–4 hr.
Aspart		"
Short-acting		
Regular	30–60 min.	4–6 hr.
Intermediate-acting		
NPH	2–4 hr.	10–16 hr.
Lente	3–4 hr.	12–18 hr.
Long-acting		
Ultralente	6–10 hr.	18–20 hr.
Glargine	4 hr.	24 hr. (no peak)

TABLE 23: ORAL HYPOGLYCEMICS

Generic Name	Brand Name	Comments
Sulfonylureas		
First generation		
Chlorpropamide	Diabinese	Long-acting agent
Tolbutamide	Orinase	
Second generation		
Glyburide	Micronase, Diabeta, Glynase	May be used as monotherapy or in combinations
Glipizide	Glucotrol, Glucotrol XL	" "
Glimepiride	Amaryl	"

Generic Name	Brand Name	Comments
Meglitinides (secretogogues)		
Repaglinide	Prandin	May be used as monotherapy or with Metformin
Nateglinide	Starlix	
Biguanides		
Metformin	Glucophage, Glucophage XR	Once-daily formulation helps with GI discomfort
Thiazolidinediones (Glitazones)		
Rosiglitazone	Avandia	Monitor liver enzymes
Pioglitazone	Actos	"
Alpha-glucosidase inhibitors		
Acarbose	Precose	Take with meal
Miglitol	Glyset	"
Combination agents		
Glyburide/Metformin	Glucovance	New combinations developed to increase patient compliance
Glipizide/Metformin	Metoglip	
Rosiglitazone/Metformin	Avandamet	" "

Infectious Diseases

TABLE 24: CEPHALOSPORINS

Generic Name	Brand Name	Route of Administration
First-generation agents		
Cefadroxil	Duricef	Oral
Cephalexin	Keflex, Keftab	Oral
Cefazolin	Ancef, Kefzol	IV, IM
Second-generation agents		
Cefaclor	Ceclor	Oral
Loracarbef	Lorabid	Oral
Cefoxitin	Mefoxin	IV
Cefuroxime	Zinacef, Ceftin	IV, IM, oral
Cefprozil	Cefzil	Oral
Third-generation agents		
Cefixime	Suprax	Oral
Ceftriaxone	Rocephin	IM, IV
Cefdinir	Omnicef	Oral
Cefpodoxime	Vantin	Oral
Cefotaxime	Claforan	IV, IM

Note: IV = intravenous; IM = intramuscular.

TABLE 25: HIV AGENTS

Generic Name	Brand Name	Comments
Reverse transcriptase inhibitors		
Nucleoside reverse transcriptase inhibitors (NRTIs)		
Zidovudine	AZT, ZDV, Retrovir	May cause severe anemia, lactic acidosis, and enlarged liver
Didanosine	ddl, Videx	Take on empty stomach May cause lactic acidosis and enlarged liver
Zalcitabine	ddC, Hivid	May cause peripheral neuropathies, lactic acidosis, and enlarged liver
Stavudine	d4T, Zerit	May cause lactic acidosis and enlarged liver
Lamivudine	3TC, Epivir	"
Abacavir	ABC, Ziagen	"
Nucleotide reverse transcriptase inhibitors		
Tenofovir	TFV, Viread	May cause lactic acidosis and enlarged liver
Non-nucleoside reverse transcriptase inhibitors (NNRTIs)		
Nevirapine	NVP, Viramune	Severe hepatotoxicity
Efavirenz	EFV, Sustiva	Dizziness, headaches
Protease inhibitors (PIs)		
Indinavir	IDV, Crixivan	Take on empty stomach
Ritonavir	RTV, Norvir	Take with food; refrigerate capsules, not solution
Nelfinavir	NFV, Viracept	Diarrhea and hyperglycemia are common side effects
Saquinavir	Invirase, Fortovase	"
Amprenavir	APV, Agenerase	Large quantities of propylene glycol in solution may cause toxicities

Antineoplastic Agents

TABLE 26: CHEMOTHERAPEUTIC AGENTS

Generic Names	Brand Names	Primary Antineoplastic Indications
Alkylating agents		
Busulfan	Myleran	Chromic myelogenous leukemia
Carboplatin	Paraplatin	Ovarian cancer, lung cancer, bladder cancer, breast cancer
Carmustine	BiCNU	Brain tumors, multiple myeloma, melanoma, lung cancer, colon cancer
Chlorambucil	Leukeran	Chronic lymphocytic leukemia, Hodgkin's and non-Hodgkin's lymphoma, breast cancer, ovarian cancer, testicular cancer
Cisplatin	Platinol, Platinol AQ	Head, neck, breast, testicular, bladder, cervical, esophageal, and ovarian cancer
Cyclophosphamide	Cytoxan, Neosar	Hodgkin's and non-Hodgkin's lymphoma, several types of leukemia, neuroblastoma, retinoblastoma
Dacarbazine	DTIC-Dome	Malignant melanoma, Hodgkin's disease, soft-tissue sarcomas, fibrosarcomas, islet cell carcinoma of the pancreas, neuroblastoma, thyroid cancer
Ifosfamide	Ifex	Lung cancer, Hodgkin's and non-Hodgkin's lymphoma, breast, ovarian, and testicular cancers, pancreatic and gastric carcinoma
Lomustine	CeeNU	Brain tumors, Hodgkin's and non-Hodgkin's lymphoma, melanoma, renal carcinoma, lung cancer, colon cancer
Mechlorethamine	Mustargen Hydrochloride	Hodgkin's and non-Hodgkin's lymphoma
Melphalan	Alkeran	Epithelial ovarian carcinoma, neuroblastoma, breast cancer
Streptozocin	Zanosar	Metastatic islet cell cancer of the pancreas, Hodgkin's disease

Generic Names	Brand Names	Primary Antine-oplastic Indications	Generic Names	Brand Names	Primary Antine-oplastic Indications
Antimetabolites			Tamoxifen	Nolvadex	Breast cancer
Cladribine	Leustatin	Hairy cell leukemia, chronic lymphocytic leukemia, non-Hodgkin's lymphomas, progressive multiple sclerosis	*Antibiotics*		
			Bleomycin	Blenoxane	Squamous cell carcinoma, melanoma, sarcomas, testicular carcinoma, Hodgkin's and non-Hodgkin's lymphoma
Cytarabine	Cutosar-U, DepoCyt	Leukemia, lymphoma, meningeal leukemia, meningeal lymphoma	Dactinomycin	Cosmegen	Testicular tumors, melanoma, choriocar-cinoma, Wilm's tumor, neuroblastoma, retinoblastoma, rhabdomyosarcoma, uterine sarcomas, Kaposi's sarcoma
Floxuridine	FUDR	Gastrointestinal adenocarcinoma metastatic to the liver			
Fludarabine	Fludara	Chronic lymphocytic leukemia			
Fluorouracil	Adrucil	Stomach, colon, rectum, breast, and pancreas cancer	Daunorubicin	Cerubidine, DaunoXome	Leukemias, lymphoma, Kaposi's sarcoma
Gemcitabine	Gemzar	Pancreatic cancer, non-small cell lung cancer	Doxorubicin	Adriamycin PFS, Adriamycin RDF, Rubex, Doxil	Leukemias; lympho-mas; multiple my-eloma; osseous and non-osseous sarcomas; mesotheliomas; germ cell tumors of the ovary or testes; carcinomas of the head, neck, thyroid, and lung; Wilm's tumor; breast, stomach, pancreas, liver, ovary, bladder, prostate, and uterine cancer; neuroblastoma
Mercaptopurine	Purinethol	Acute leukemias			
Methotrexate	Folex PFS	Trophoblastic neo-plasms; leukemias, breast, head, neck, stomach, esophagus, testicular, and lung cancers; osteosarcoma			
Hormones					
Diethystilbestrol	Stilphosteral	Metastatic prostatic carcinoma and postmenopausal inoperable, progressing breast cancer	Idarubicin	Idamycin	Acute myeloid leukemia, acute lymphocytic leukemia in children
Estramustine	Emcyt	Prostatic carcinoma	Mitomycin	Mutamycin	Adenocarcinoma of the stomach or pancreas, bladder cancer, colorectal cancer
Flutamide	Eulexin	Metastatic prostatic carcinoma			
Letrozole	Femara	Advanced postmeno-pausal breast cancer	Mitoxantrone	Novantrone	Acute nonlymphocytic leukemia, various other leukemias, lymphoma, breast cancer
Leuprolide	Lupron, Lupron Depot, Lupron Depot-3 Month, Lupron Depot-4 Month, Lupron Depot-Ped	Advanced prostatic cancer, endometriosis, central precocious puberty			
			Mitotic inhibitors		
Medroxypro-gesterone	Curretab, Cycrin, Depo-Provera, Provera	Endometrial cancer	Docetaxel	Taxotere	Breast cancer, non-small lung cancer; under investigation for treatment of gastric, pancreatic, head and neck, and ovarian cancers, among others
Megestrol acetate	Megace	Breast and endometrial carcinoma			

Generic Names	Brand Names	Primary Antine-oplastic Indications
Etoposide	Toposar, VePesid	Lymphomas, leukemias, lung, testicular, bladder, and prostate carcinomas; hepatoma; rhab-domyosarcoma; uterine carcinoma; neuroblastoma; Kaposi's sarcoma
Paclitaxel	Paxene, Taxol	Ovarian carcinoma, breast cancer, non-small cell lung cancer, Kaposi's sarcoma
Vinblastine	Alkaban-AQ, Velban	Hodgkin's and non-Hodgkin's lymphoma; testicular, lung, head and neck, breast, and renal carcinomas; Kaposi's sarcoma; choriocarcinoma
Vincristine	Oncovin, Vincasar PFS	Leukemias, Hodgkin's and non-Hodgkin's lymphoma, Wilm's tumor, neuroblastoma, rhabdomyosarcoma
Vinorelbine	Navelbine	Non-small cell lung cancer

Miscellaneous agents

Generic Names	Brand Names	Primary Antine-oplastic Indications
Asparaginase	Elspar	Acute lymphocytic leukemia, lymphoma
Dacarbazine	DTIC-Dome	Malignant melanoma, Hodgkin's disease, soft-tissue sarcomas, fibrosarcomas, rhabdomyosarcoma, islet cell carcinoma of the pancreas, medullary carcinoma of the thyroid, neuroblastoma
Hydroxyurea	Droxia, Hydrea	Chronic myelogenous leukemia; brain tumors; head and neck tumors; uterine, cervical, and non-small cell lung cancers
Interferon alpha 2a	Roferon-A	Hairy cell leukemia, Kaposi's sarcoma, chronic myelogenous leukemia

Generic Names	Brand Names	Primary Antine-oplastic Indications
Interferon alpha 2b	Intron-A	Hairy cell leukemia, malignant melanoma, Kaposi's sarcoma, follicular non-Hodgkin's lymphoma
Procarbazine	Matulane	Hodgkin's and non-Hodgkin's lymphoma, brain tumor, bron-chogenic carcinoma

Topical Medications

Ophthalmic Medications

TABLE 27: OPHTHALMIC AGENTS		
Generic Name	Brand Name	Dosage Forms
Antibiotic agents		
Gentamicin		Solution, ointment
Tobramycin	Tobrex	Solution, ointment
Na sulfacetamide	Sulf-10	Solution, ointment
Ciprofloxacin	Ciloxan	Solution
Ofloxacin	Ocuflox	Solution
Levofloxacin	Quixin	Solution
Norfloxacin	Chibroxin	Solution
Combination agents		
Neomycin/Polymixin/ Hydrcortisone	Cortisporin	Solution, ointment
Neomycin/Polymixin/ Dexamethasone	Maxitrol	Solution, ointment
Tobramycin/ Dexamethasone	Tobradex	Solution, ointment
Antiviral agents		
Vidarabine	Vira-A	Ointment
Trifluridine	Viroptic	Solution
Ganciclovir	Vitrasert	Implant
Idoxuridine	Herplex	Solution
Antihistamine/decongestant agents		
Lodoxamide	Alomide	Solution
Levocabastine	Livostin	Solution
Ketotifen	Zaditor	Solution
Olopatadine	Patanol	Solution
Emedastine	Emadine	Solution
Azelastine	Optivar	Solution

Generic Name	Brand Name	Dosage Forms
Antiglaucoma agents		
Beta-blockers		
Betaxolol	Betoptic, Betoptic-S	Solution, suspension
Carteolol	Ocupress	Solution
Levobunolol	Betagan	Solution
Timolol	Timoptic, Timoptic-XE	Solution
Carbonic anhydrase inhibitors		
Dorzolamide	Trusopt	Solution
Brinzolamide	Azopt	Solution
Prostaglandin analog		
Lotanoprost	Xalatan	Solution

Otic Medications

TABLE 28: COMMON INGREDIENTS IN OTIC MEDICATIONS

Ingredient	Indication
Acetic acid	Antibacterial
Aluminum acetate	Antibacterial
Antipyrine	Analgesic
Benzalkonium chloride	Antiseptic
Benzethonium chloride	Antiseptic
Benzocaine	Anesthetic
Boric acid	Drying agent for auditory canal
Chloramphenicol	Antibacterial
Ciprofloxacin	Antibacterial
Hydrocortisone	Corticosteroid
M-cresyl acetate	Antibacterial
Neomycin	Antibacterial
Polymyxin B	Antibacterial

Intranasal Products

TABLE 29: INTRANASAL FORMULATIONS

Generic Name	Brand Name	Onset of Action
Antihistamines		
Azelastine	Astelin	Immediate
Corticosteroids		
Beclomethasone diproprionate	Beconase, Vancenase, Beconase AQ, Vancenase AQ	Few days to 2 weeks " " "
Budesonide	Rhinocort, Rhinocort AQ	24 hrs. "
Flunisolide	Nasalide, Nasarel	Few days to 2 weeks
Fluticasone	Flonase	Few days
Mometasone	Nasonex	2 days
Triamcinolone acetonide	Nasacort, Nasacort AQ	12 hrs. to a few days "
Mast cell stabilizers		
Cromolyn sodium	Nasalcrom	1 to 2 weeks
Topical decongestants		
Oxymetazoline	Neo-Synephrine - 12-hour Duration Afrin -12-hour Dristan -12-hour Nostrilla -12-hour	Immediate " " " "
Xylometazoline	Otrivin Natru-Vent	Immediate "
Naphazoline	Privine	Immediate

Dermatological Agents

TABLE 30: TOPICAL AGENTS

Generic Name	Trade Name	Dosage Forms
Low-potency corticosteroids		
Desonide	DesOwen	Cream, ointment, gel, spray
Hydrocortisone	Various brands	Cream, ointment, gel, spray, solution, lotion
Medium-potency corticosteroids		
Hydrocortisone valerate	Westcort	Cream, ointment
Mometasone	Elocon	Cream, ointment, lotion
High-potency corticosteroids		
Betamethasone diproprionate	Diprosone	Cream, ointment, lotion
Betamethasone	Valerate	Ointment
Desoximetasone	Topicort	Cream, ointment, gel
Fluocinolone	Synalar	Cream, ointment
Fluocinonide	Lidex	Cream, ointment, gel
Halcinonide	Halog	Cream, ointment
Triamcinolone	Aristocort	Cream, ointment, lotion

Generic Name	Trade Name	Dosage Forms
Very high potency corticosteroids		
Clobetasol	Temovate, Embeline, Cormax	Cream, ointment "
Diflorasone	Psorcon-E	Cream, ointment (emollient)
Halobetasol	Ultravate	Cream, ointment
Augmented betamethasone diproprionate	Diprolene	Cream, ointment
Topical antifungals		
Clotrimazole	Lotrimin AF, Mycelex	Cream, lotion, solution
Miconazole	Micatin, Desenex	Cream, powder, spray
Terbinafine	Lamisil AT	Cream
Tolnaftate	Tinactin, Aftate	Cream, solution, powder, aerosol
Ketoconazole	Nizoral	Cream, shampoo
Naftifine	Naftin	Cream, gel
Econazole	Spectazole	Cream

Nutritional Products

TABLE 31: VITAMINS		
Common Name	**Chemical Name**	**Type (fat-soluble versus water-soluble)**
Vitamin A	Retinol	Fat-soluble
Vitamin B_1	Thiamine	Water-soluble
Vitamin B_2	Riboflavin	Water-soluble
Vitamin B_3	Niacin, Nicotinic Acid	Water-soluble
Vitamin B_5	Pantothenic Acid	Water-soluble
Vitamin B_6	Pyridoxine	Water-soluble
Vitamin B_{12}	Cyanocobalamine	Water-soluble
Vitamin C	Ascorbic Acid	Water-soluble
Vitamin D	Ergocalciferol	Fat-soluble
Vitamin E	Tocopherol	Fat-soluble
Vitamin K	Phytonadione	Fat-soluble

TABLE 32: MINERALS AND THEIR FUNCTIONS IN THE BODY		
Mineral	**Amount Present in Body**	**Function**
Calcium	Major element	Important in bone and tooth formation and in nerve function

Mineral	Amount Present in Body	Function
Chloride	Major element	Used in the production of hydrochloric acid; closely connected with sodium in body tissues, fluids, and excretions
Chromium	Trace element	A co-factor for insulin
Copper	Trace element	Important for hemoglobin
Fluoride	Trace element	Associated with tooth enamel
Iodine	Trace element	Linked with thyroid function
Iron	Trace element	Important part of the hemoglobin molecule and required in many enzymes
Magnesium	Major element	Second most abundant mineral found in the body; important in body enzymes and in nerve and muscle function
Manganese	Trace element	Needed for growth as well as for various enzymes
Phosphorous	Major element	Important in metabolism and acid-base regulation
Potassium	Major element	Primary mineral found inside cells; important in cellular metabolism and in nerve and muscle function
Selenium	Trace element	Important in cellular metabolism
Sodium	Major element	Important in growth and in muscle function
Sulfur	Major element	Important for many proteins and heparin
Zinc	Trace element	Important for growth and for insulin utilization

Suggested Reading*

Basic and clinical pharmacology, 6th ed. Norwalk, CT: Appleton & Lange; 1995.

Facts and comparisons. St. Louis, MO: Facts and Comparisons, Inc.

Merck manual of diagnosis and therapy, 16th ed., Rahway, NJ: Merck Research Laboratories; 1992.

USP DI, Volume I, drug information for the health care professional. Rockville, MD: United States Pharmacopeia Convention, Inc.; 1997.

USP DI, Volume II, advice for the patient. Rockville, MD: United States Pharmacopeia Convention, Inc.; 1997.

Des Prez RM, Heim CR. Mycobacterium tuberculosis. In: Mandell GL, Douglas RG, Bennett JE, eds. Principles and practice of infectious diseases. New York: Churchill Livingstone, Inc; 1990:1877–82.

Footnotes

* See chapter 7 for more information about medication references.

" Marks are used in table columns to signify repeated application of previous information.

,

Self-Assessment Questions

1. Which drug belongs to the class of calcium channel blockers?
   a. Lidocaine
   b. Calcium carbonate
   c. Nicardipine
   d. Loperidine
   e. Meperidine

2. Which of the following is *not* an opiate analgesic?
   a. Ibuprofen
   b. Hydrocodone
   c. Morphine
   d. Codeine
   e. Hydromorphone

3. Which of the following may be used as antineoplastic agents?
   a. Docetaxel
   b. Doxorubicin
   c. Medroxyprogesterone
   d. Gemcitabine
   e. All of the above

4. Which of the following is *not* a trace element?
   a. Iron
   b. Potassium
   c. Selenium
   d. Chromium
   e. Copper

5. The brand name for cefoxitin is:
   a. Ancef
   b. Rocephin
   c. Fortaz
   d. Mefoxin
   e. Cefizox

6. Which of the following is a diuretic?
   a. Hydroxyzine
   b. Hydrochlorothiazide
   c. Hydroxyurea
   d. Hydrocortisone
   e. Hydrochloric acid

7. Which of the following is *not* used to treat diabetes?
   a. Insulin
   b. Glyburide
   c. Metformin
   d. Metolazone
   e. Pioglitazone

8. Which of the following is the brand name for meperidine?
   a. Demerol
   b. Lasix
   c. Lanoxin
   d. Vicodin
   e. Dilaudid

9. Which of the following is Vitamin B_1?
   a. Folic acid
   b. Riboflavin
   c. Thiamine
   d. Ascorbic acid
   e. Nicotinic acid

10. Which antihistamine is available without a prescription?
    a. Loratidine
    b. Diphenhydramine
    c. Chlorpheniramine
    d. Clemastine
    e. All of the above

Self-Assessment Answers

1. c
2. a
3. e
4. b
5. d
6. b
7. d
8. a
9. c
10. e

How to Take a Test

NANCY F. FJORTOFT, KRISTIN LANGE

You are not alone if you face upcoming examinations with dread and anxiety. Most people do. But exams serve a purpose. They are intended to test your knowledge, not your patience and endurance. Tests are helpful to others who are attempting to determine your understanding and knowledge of specific areas. Tests also help you to understand what areas you are competent in and what areas you need to focus on in terms of your own learning and development.

This chapter reviews preparation tips and test-taking strategies. It concludes with a section on how to deal with the anxiety most of us feel prior to an examination.

Written Examinations

There are two basic kinds of written examinations. The first is the objective examination. Objective examinations include multiple-choice, true/false, and matching questions. Objective examinations are designed to test your ability to recognize, rather than recall, facts and information. The second type is the essay examination. Essay examinations are tests for which respondents give long, written answers. They provide the opportunity for respondents to organize their knowledge, integrate materials, and express themselves. The two kinds of tests require different skill sets. Because your exam will be objective multiple choice, this chapter focuses on techniques to help you perform at your best on this type of examination.

Multiple-Choice Questions

A multiple-choice question normally begins with an incomplete sentence or question, known as a *stem*. The stem is followed by a series of choices for completing the sentence or answering the question, known as *responses*. The responses are usually lettered *a*, *b*, *c*, and *d*. Typically, there are four, sometimes five, responses to choose from. You complete the sentence or answer the question by choosing the correct or best response. For example, a typical multiple-choice question will look like this:

Learning Objectives

After completing this chapter, the technician should be able to

1. Discuss basic study and review skills for objective tests.

2. List basic strategies for taking objective tests.

3. Define common trouble areas in taking objective tests and describe how to manage these difficulties.

4. Recognize test anxiety and define common relaxation techniques.

(Stem) The capital of Illinois is:

(Responses)

a. Springfield
b. Chicago
c. Rockford
d. St. Louis

Normally, the directions are to pick the one best response. However, the directions vary, so read the directions and the stem carefully. You may be instructed to pick the incorrect option or to pick more than one option. There are also questions that present the stem as a complete statement. Key words to note in the stem are the subject of the question and any qualifiers or adjectives that further define the best answer.

Preparing for Objective Exams

You may be fresh out of the classroom with recent experience in preparing for and taking objective exams, or you might not have taken an exam in quite some time. Whatever the case, it's always useful to review good study skills. This section reviews some basic study and test preparation techniques.

Planning Ahead

The first step in preparing for an exam is to check the date, time, and place of the exam. Mark your calendar and take the time to find the location in advance. You do not want to be late for the exam because you got lost. Estimate how long it will take you to get to the test center. You may even want to do a test drive. Find out where parking is available, or make a trial run on public transportation.

Make sure you understand the scope of the exam. In other words, how long is the exam, and what material will it cover? What materials, if any, can you bring with you? Are you allowed to use a calculator or supplemental resources? Do you need number 2 pencils? Make sure you understand the purpose and format of the test.

Time Management

Every busy person needs a schedule. But before you can plan your study schedule, you first need a thorough understanding of how you study. Answer these basic questions about yourself:

When is the best time of day for me to study?

How do I best learn?

If you are unsure of the answers to these questions, you may want to monitor yourself for a week. Develop a time chart, and follow your activities. Are there any times of the day when you are more productive than others? Think about how you learn as well. What tasks help you learn? Do you learn best by doing or by reading? Some people find reading aloud to be a helpful memorization technique. This kind of self-knowledge will guide you in developing your study schedule. Even though family and work responsibilities may take most of your time, try to use your most productive time of the day for your studies.

Think in small increments of time. Do not postpone studying because you do not have all afternoon to devote to your studies. Plan and organize small learning tasks that can occur in short blocks of time. It is easier to learn when you break your studies into smaller increments.[1] For example, each of these is an increment: review your notes, generate questions from your notes, make a question chart (more on that later) or key word list, and define key words. Don't postpone your studies while you wait for that perfect free day. That free day may not come.

Using Question Charts

One study technique that has been found to be useful in organizing and learning information is a question chart.[1] Question charts help you make connections between information that is new to you and what you already know—an important step in the learning process. For example, your topic is medication administration. **Table 6-1** gives an example of how to set up your chart.

Make question charts to cover all the main concepts in this review guide. Complete the charts as you read, revising and adding questions as you go, and then use them as study guides.

Defining Terms

Make a separate section in your notes for terms and their definitions. Define each term by a key word or phrase. Review those terms every day, and add terms to your list as you read new material. This is an example of one of the small learning tasks discussed earlier.

Group Review

Some people find it helpful to meet with other students to review notes, ask questions, and compare perceptions. This may or may not be helpful to you; it all depends on your personal style. If you do study with

TABLE 6-1. SAMPLE QUESTION CHART

Medication Administration

Questions	Intravenous	Oral	Topical
What are the available dosage forms?	Solutions, Suspensions	Tablets, Capsules, Solutions, Suspensions, Powders	Ointments, Creams, Patches
What are the advantages of this administration?	Quick onset of action	Convenience	Limited systemic route of absorption (ointments and creams only)
What are the disadvantages of this route of administration?	No drug recall Pain at injection site	Slower onset of action Taste, palatability	Inconvenience

others, have an organized agenda so that time is not wasted. Listen and learn from your colleagues, but if you are unsure, check your references. Do not take another person's word for something you are not sure of. Look it up.

Mock Exams

Use your question charts to make up your own exam, or if you are working with a group of colleagues, write questions for each other. This is often a helpful way to prepare for exams. The practice exam included in this book is a good way to test your comprehension of the material.

Final Review

Suppose the test is tomorrow. Spend your final review time reviewing, reciting, and summarizing your notes. When you are reviewing your term list or mastering your notes, make sure that you review from both directions. Begin first with the most difficult material, or reverse the review process by rearranging your notes, reviewing from back to front, and beginning in the middle. Don't get tied to order. If there is anything you are not certain of, now is the time to look it up and learn it. Recite from your summary sheets.

Personal Preparation

Now that you are mentally prepared, prepare yourself physically for your exam. Go to your exam rested. You will not do well on your exam if you are so sleepy that you cannot concentrate on the questions. Eat a good breakfast before your exam. It's hard for the mind to concentrate if the body is demanding attention. Your brain functions better with a supply of energy. Also, it is probably not wise to start a new diet, quit smoking, or begin a new exercise regimen until after you complete the exam. You need to focus your energies on preparing for and taking the exam, not on redesigning your lifestyle.

Prepare emotionally as well. Remember that the purpose of this exam is not to fail you or to humiliate you, but to assist you professionally. So relax, be prepared, and concentrate. With preparation and strategy on your side, you will perform at your best.

Taking Objective Exams

You've been preparing for weeks and now the big test date has finally arrived. This section outlines several steps and strategies that are useful in successfully completing an objective test.

Come Prepared

The first step in successfully taking objective tests is to come prepared. By now you should understand the purpose of the test, the format, and the length of time you are allowed to complete the test. Make sure you bring the supplies you need to take the test: pencils, erasers, and a calculator if allowed.

Arrive at the test site 30 to 40 minutes early. This will allow you time to find the restrooms, get a good seat where you can see the clock and the blackboard, and get comfortable. Make sure the surroundings are adequate in your chosen seat location. Is there enough light for you to read the exam? Are there any distracting noises? Everyone has a different threshold of distraction. For example, you may find the ticking of a clock absolutely maddening. Understand what distracts you, and make sure you are in a good location in the room to prevent distractions.

Test-Taking Strategies

Some basic strategies are helpful to most people taking objective tests. The first thing every test taker should do is to look over the test carefully. Check to make sure that you have all the pages. The minute or two you spend looking through the test will help you make better use of time and improve your test performance.

The second step is to use your time wisely. Set yourself a schedule. Using your time wisely is dependent on reviewing the test carefully. The only way to plan your time is to be aware of how many and what types of questions you must answer. You should have an idea at what time you should be halfway done the exam. For example, if you have 2 hours for a test, you should be at least halfway through it by the end of the first hour. Remember to leave extra time for particularly tough questions and for review. Work as rapidly as possible with reasonable assurance of accuracy.

The third strategy is to read carefully. This includes both the directions and the questions.

■ Do you answer the questions on the exam itself or on the answer sheet?

■ Can you use ink or only pencil? If you are using an answer sheet, most likely you will need to use a pencil.

■ How long do you have to complete the test? If you are unsure, ask the proctor. Never, never be in doubt.

Sections of the exam may vary, so take the time to read the directions carefully at the beginning of each new section, and keep those directions in mind while answering the questions. Making careless mistakes because you misunderstood the directions is not an effective test-taking strategy! For example, the directions may read, "select the incorrect response," or "mark the two best answers."

Part of reading carefully involves reading the questions as they are, not as you would like them to be. In other words, don't look for answers you have memorized. Answer the question. Many people find it helpful to mark the key words in the stem so they do not forget them or misinterpret them. Also look for and mark the question words. This will help you answer the question as written. Some common question words are *what*, *how*, *when*, and *define*.

A fourth strategy is to leave your assumptions at home. You should not anticipate or assume trick questions. For example, you may know the correct answer is *d*, but you feel you have already answered too many questions with *d*. Take the question at face value and mark the answer you think is correct. Also, do not assume that methods or procedures that you use at work are necessarily the correct ones. "Because that's the way we do it around here" may not be based on fact or best practice.

Going through the test at least two or even three times is another strategy for successful test taking. Go through the test completely the first time and answer all the "easy" questions that you are sure of. While you are doing the first run-through, mark the questions you need to come back to with a circle. By answering all the easy questions first, you can be assured that you have answered the questions that you know. This strategy also builds confidence. In the stem of one question, you may also find an answer to another question.

On the second run-through, answer the questions that you are unsure of by considering all the alternatives and eliminating the options that you know are inappropriate or incorrect. Relate the remaining options to the stem and balance them against each other. Use the information obtained from other questions to help you.

On the third run-through, look at the remaining questions. If it is in your best interest to guess, do so. Always guess if your chances of gaining points are greater than your chances of losing points. Use the following strategies for intelligent guessing:

■ The most general option is often the correct one because it allows for exceptions. If three of the four options are specific in nature and one is more general, choose the more general option.

■ The correct choice is most often a middle value. If the options range in value (for example, from high to low or from big to small), then eliminate the extreme values and choose from the middle values.

■ The longest option is often the correct one. If three options are much shorter than the fourth, then choose the longest answer.

■ When two options have opposite meanings, then the correct answer is usually one of these.

■ Look for grammatical agreement between the stem and the answers. For example, if the stem uses a singular verb tense, then the answer should also be singular. Eliminate the answers that don't produce grammatically correct sentences. Most multiple-choice questions are designed as sentence completions.[2]

Computerized Testing

Computerized testing poses a unique set of problems. People vary in their level of comfort in dealing with computer programs. If you are not accustomed to working on a computer, it would be wise to complete a practice exam in that format prior to the actual test if possible. The Pharmacy Technician Certification Board also sells a practice exam on its Web page (www.ptcb.org). Other programs with computerized standardized tests are available commercially, such as SAT practice programs. These tests may give you practice in computerized testing formats, although the questions will not relate to the Pharmacy Technician Certification Exam.

Computerized tests often employ many of the same types of questions and question formats as paper tests, and you should use most of the same strategies, such as reading both the questions and the answers carefully. One thing that is very different is that your ability to go back and review previous questions is often limited or completely prohibited. It is important for you to try to pace yourself accordingly. Try to make your best answer in the time available to you and move on to the next question. If you are, in fact, able to move backward through the test or parts of it, then you may choose to go back and review your answers. Whether or not this is an option will be made clear in the instructions for the test. If you have a question about looking at already answered questions that is not dealt with in the instructions, you should ask the testing center moderator for additional information. Scratch paper is generally provided in computerized tests, but calculators are not, and you should bring your own to use during the test, as well as several sharpened number 2 pencils to write notes or work problems on the scratch paper.

Trouble Areas in Objective Exams

A couple of areas are problematic for most people taking objective exams. This section discusses those areas and provides you with some advice on tackling those obstacles.

The first potential problem area deals with specific determiners. There are positive and negative specific determiners. Positive specific determiners include *all, every, everybody, everyone, always, all the time, invariably, will certainly, will definitely, will absolutely,* and *the best.* Negative specific determiners include *none, not one, nobody, no one, never, at no time, will certainly not, will definitely not, will absolutely not, the worst,* and *impossible.* When specific determiners like these are included in an option, that option is *usually incorrect.* These words make statements absolute, and there are few absolutes in the world.[3]

However, some specific determiners are associated with correct statements. Look for more general terms such as *often, perhaps, seldom, generally, may,* and *usually.* Life more often reflects statements that use these kinds of

words, rather than the absolute terms presented in the previous paragraph. When you are reading the question, circle the specific determiner so that you keep careful track of them. Don't ignore them when answering the question.

The second problem area deals with negative terms. It is more difficult to interpret statements that contain negatives than it is to interpret statements without negatives. Here's an example of a double-negative statement: "Donald works well with patients. Therefore it is not untrue to say that he may be a good pharmacy technician." Cross out the *not* and the *un-* and reread the statement. It means the same thing, but is easier to understand. Negatives include words such as *no, not, none,* and *never,* and prefixes such as *il-, un-,* and *im-.* Negative prefixes are particularly difficult because they are easily overlooked when reading a statement. Underline negatives in the question so that you do not overlook them when answering the question.[3]

Another common trouble area in objective tests is "all or none of the above" questions. One way to confirm the choice of "all of the above" is to find two correct answers among the options. For example, if you are confident that two of the four options are correct, then choosing "all of the above" is a pretty safe bet. Similarly, if you find one that is definitely incorrect, the "all of the above" must be ruled out.

The last type of question that is usually problematic for test takers is the best choice option. The options presented may not contain the correct answer, but instead options from which you choose the best. Another way of thinking of it is to think of the correct option as the least problematic. Select your answer by a process of elimination.[3]

Mental Blocks

You know you know the material. You've been answering questions—and all of a sudden, you can't seem to think. You have a mental block. One useful technique is to think of the multiple-choice question as a series of true and false statements. In other words, make statements or complete sentences out of each of the options and then ask yourself if the statement is true or false. This change in perspective may help you to answer a difficult question or just refresh your thinking processes. However, keep your time limitations in mind and don't spend too much time on any one question. Skip difficult questions and come back to them, or take a quick 1-minute mental break to refresh yourself.

Final Review

Always plan on saving time to review your test before handing it in to the proctor. Check your math if any of the questions required calculations. Check your answer sheet if you are using one. Are all the bubbles filled in completely? And most important, check your answers. Contrary to popular belief, research has shown that test takers generally increase their scores when they review their answers and make changes.[4] Make changes thoughtfully, though. When changing an answer, make sure you have taken into consideration the reasons why you answered the questions the way you did in the first place.

Finally, don't let other test takers distract you; concentrate on what you are doing. Do not be concerned if other people are finishing the exam before you. They may be finishing early because they simply are not as prepared as you are and therefore cannot answer all the questions. There is little relationship between the amount of time spent on a test and the test scores.

Coping with Text Anxieties

At the beginning of this chapter, we discussed how many people face taking an exam with dread and anxiety. It has been estimated that half of the nation's students suffer test anxiety, and one-quarter of them are significantly hampered by it.[5] You may feel faint at heart, apprehensive, nervous, nauseated, or dizzy, or you may even have heart palpitations. Some people describe it as "my mind goes blank." Some amount of test anxiety is normal, so you just need to learn how to make it work for you. The first step is to recognize that some anxiety is natural; it serves as a primary motivator in your performance.

There are three components of test anxiety. The first one is fear of failure. Nobody likes to fail, but remember to keep it in perspective. Tests just measure and assess one aspect of your life. Passing or failing a test reflects your performance in one area at one particular time. The second component of test anxiety is the pressure of time. You have a limited amount of time to accomplish a task and to accomplish the task as accurately as possible. We all feel the pressure of time in many situations aside from testing. The third component is the logistics of taking the exam. You must read the instructions, follow them, understand the questions, and select the correct answer. Generally, the higher the stakes, the more anxiety you may feel, particularly if the competition is intense.[5]

If your anxiety is moderate, several relaxation techniques are helpful in calming your nerves. Physical relaxation is one technique. First, sit comfortably with both feet on the floor and your hands resting on your thighs. Release all your body tension and close your eyes and count backward from 10 to 1. Count only on each exhalation and breathe very deeply from the abdomen.[1]

Another physical technique is to clench your hands tightly for 5 to 10 seconds and then slowly relax your hands. Repeat this process throughout the muscles in your entire body. Complete your relaxation exercise by taking a deep breath and tensing your entire body, then relaxing it.

Now that your body is relaxed, try to relax your mind as well. One popular technique is imagining yourself in a peaceful setting. Picture a pleasing situation, such as lying on a favorite beach, sitting in your backyard with the sun shining, or taking a walk in a park or along the lake. When you are feeling particularly stressed, imagine peaceful images.

At all costs, avoid fear-generating thoughts. Do not focus on the negative consequences; instead, focus on the positive outcomes of your examination.

These are just a few simple techniques that may help you relax so you can do your best. For some, however, test anxiety is so severe that it prevents them from performing at their best. If you experience severe anxiety, you may benefit from seeking personal counseling.

Conclusion

Now that the exam is over, you deserve a reward. Be kind to yourself. However, do spend a few minutes to review what worked for you and what didn't. Think about your preparation. Did you allow yourself enough time? Did you understand what was important to study and learn, and what were minor details? How about the test itself? Did you overview the test, run through it several times, and save time for review and checking your answers? One of the most important lessons in life is to learn from your experiences, so evaluate your performance and learn how you can make it better. You may register and take this examination again if you need to. Most likely, there will be other exams in your life as well.

This chapter presented an overview of objective tests, basic study skills, and test-taking strategies. It also presented some simple techniques for relaxation to refresh you. But remember, no matter how effective the strategies, there is no substitute for adequate and thorough preparation. Begin your preparation early, be organized, use small increments of time, break your studying down into small tasks, and relax.

References

1. Heiman M, Slomianko J. *Success in College and Beyond.* Allston, MA: Learning to Learn Inc.; 1992.

2. Pauk W. *How to Study in College.* 5th ed. Boston: Houghton Mifflin; 1993.

3. Shepherd JF. *College Study Skills.* 2nd ed. Boston: Houghton Mifflin; 1983.

4. Millman J, Pauk W. *How to Take Tests.* New York: McGraw-Hill; 1969.

5. Hill KT. Interfering effects of test anxiety on test performance: a growing educational problem and solutions to it. *Ill Sch Res Dev.* 1983;20:8–19.

Practice Exam

Choose the *one* best answer for each of the following questions.

1. Information that is *not* generally found in a patient's profile in an outpatient pharmacy includes which of the following?
   a. preferences regarding child-resistant packaging
   b. date of birth
   c. preferred hospital
   d. prescription and refill history
   e. allergies

2. Which of the following *is not* a part of a syringe?
   a. plunger
   b. Luer-lok tip
   c. bevel
   d. barrel
   e. calibration marks

3. Which abbreviation is *not* used to specify a unit of measure?
   a. hx
   b. oz
   c. kg
   d. ml
   e. tsp

4. What is the *inventory par level?*
   a. the amount of drug that should be purchased at one time
   b. the inventory level at which an order should be placed to prevent running too low
   c. the maximum amount of a particular drug that should be on the shelf at any time
   d. the number generally posted on the shelf label where the drug is stored
   e. b and d

5. Express the following in reduced form: 3/4 + 7/8
   a. 13/8
   b. 2
   c. 1 3/8

d. 1.5

e. 1 5/8

6. A child is to be treated with 50 milligrams (mg) of a particular drug per kilograms (kg) of body weight. If the child weighs 38 pounds, what is the dose of the drug that should be administered (round to the nearest 5 mg)?

a. 430 mg

b. 865 mg

c. 1,200 mg

d. 1,655 mg

e. 1,900 mg

7. Using the information from the previous question, how much would be needed to provide the correct dose if the drug concentration is 100 mg per milliliter (ml)?

a. 4.3 ml

b. 8.65 ml

c. 12 ml

d. 16.55 ml

e. 19 ml

8. Which of the following is *not* a low molecular weight heparin (LMWH)?

a. heparin

b. enoxaparin

c. dalteparin

d. tinzaparin

e. All of the above are LMWHs.

9. A medication order should contain all of the following elements *except* which one?

a. the dosage form of the product to be dispensed

b. the patient's room number

c. the name of the drug

d. the dose of the drug

e. All of the above should be included.

10. What is *quality control*?

a. a final check to ensure safety and quality of the preparation

b. something done only by the pharmacist

c. something accomplished by comparing the finished product with pictures of what it should look like

d. all of the above

e. none of the above

11. Which of the following should be used to clean the interior of the laminar flow hood?

a. 70 percent isopropyl alcohol

b. 98 percent ethyl alcohol

c. water and a lint-free cloth

d. 50 percent acetone

e. a and c

12. Which of the following is (are) used to describe a needle?

a. bevel

b. shaft length

c. gauge

d. all of the above

e. none of the above

13. Which statement(s) is (are) true of the Internet?

a. It contains only reputable sources.

b. It can be used to access on-line versions of many of the popular print references.

c. It should be recommended to computer-using patients instead of offering patient counseling.

d. It is a good place to look for general information about diseases, such as contacting support groups.

e. b and d

14. Which abbreviation stands for "before meals"?

a. hs

b. pc

c. tid

d. qd

e. ac

15. Which of the following is *false* concerning the drug receiving process in a pharmacy?

a. It is not necessary to verify the number of boxes delivered.

b. Each item should be carefully checked to make sure it is the correct drug and correct strength.

c. Expiration dating should be checked so that short-dated products can be returned.

d. Controlled substances require additional record-keeping steps.

e. The person who checked in the order should sign the invoice or packing slip.

16. Which of the following is *false* regarding the Poison Prevention Packaging Act?

a. A patient may opt out of the requirements of the act upon request.
b. The act requires all prescriptions to be dispensed in child-resistant packaging, with a few exceptions.
c. One exception to the act is nitroglycerin tablets.
d. A physician specializing in geriatrics may instruct a pharmacy never to use child-resistant packages for any of his prescriptions because all his patients are elderly.
e. The act does not apply to hospital dispensing for inpatients.

17. What is 1 kg equal to?
    a. 1,000 mg
    b. 2.2 pounds
    c. 10,000 mcg
    d. all of the above
    e. none of the above

18. A patient is supposed to take 375 mg of an antibiotic three times daily for 10 days. The pharmacy dispenses 250 mg per 5 ml suspension. How much must the patient take per dose?
    a. 3.75 ml
    b. 5 ml
    c. 7.5 ml
    d. 8.75 ml
    e. 10 ml

19. Using the information from the previous question, how much should the pharmacy dispense for the full 10-day supply?
    a. 100 ml
    b. 150 ml
    c. 200 ml
    d. 225 ml
    e. 300 ml

20. Which of the following is an anticonvulsant?
    a. phenytoin
    b. dexamethasone
    c. amiodarone
    d. hydrochlorothiazide
    e. albuterol

21. Which of the following is *not* used for HIV?
    a. Didanosine

b. Zidovudine
c. Nelfinavir
d. Indinavir
e. Irbesartan

22. A prescription for a controlled substance includes the DEA number BB1197967. Which of the following is *false* about the DEA number?
    a. The formula for verifying that the DEA number is correct includes adding the first, third, and fifth digits in the number.
    b. The individual to whom this number belongs has a last name that starts with a *B*.
    c. The formula for verifying that the DEA number is correct includes adding the second, fourth, and sixth digits in the number and multiplying by 2.
    d. This number must belong to a pharmacy because it begins with a *B*.
    e. This DEA number is valid.

23. Risks of intravenous (IV) therapy include which of the following?
    a. infection
    b. bleeding
    c. extravasation
    d. air embolus
    e. all of the above

24. Which is the best reference to use to look up whether an IV drug is compatible with a fluid?
    a. Drug Facts and Comparisons
    b. Red Book
    c. The Physicians' Desk Reference
    d. American Drug Index
    e. Trissel's *Handbook on Injectable Drugs*

25. Which abbreviation stands for "at bedtime"?
    a. dx
    b. ac
    c. qid
    d. hs
    e. po

26. Which question can a technician answer without involving a pharmacist?
    a. "What is the dose of morphine for a 2-year-old?"
    b. "Is phenytoin compatible with D_5W?"

c. "I have been feeling dizzy since I started my new medication. Is it possible the drug is causing this feeling?"

d. "Can I get a TB test if I am pregnant?"

e. "Is Nuprin® the same thing as ibuprofen?"

27. *Maximizing inventory turns* is which of the following?
   a. a means of minimizing inventory carrying costs
   b. rotating inventory regularly to prevent outdating
   c. the same thing as EOQ
   d. also known as the Minimum Cost Quantity Approach
   e. none of the above

28. Which Controlled Substance Schedule denotes a drug with high abuse potential and no recognized medical use?
   a. Schedule I
   b. Schedule II
   c. Schedule III
   d. Schedule IV
   e. Schedule V

29. Which of the following is true regarding a power of attorney (POA) to sign a DEA form 222?
   a. The POA can only be assigned to a pharmacist.
   b. The POA can only be assigned to one other person besides the individual whose name is on the license.
   c. The POA must be the pharmacist-in-charge.
   d. The person who signed the original license application can revoke the POA at any time.
   e. It is illegal to assign the POA to anyone to sign the DEA form 222.

30. Which of the following requires technicians to maintain confidentiality of medical information?
   a. the Food, Drug, and Cosmetic Act
   b. the Omnibus Reconciliation Act of 1990
   c. the Health Insurance Portability and Accountability Act of 1996
   d. the Federal Controlled Substance Act
   e. the Poison Prevention Packaging Act

31. What is 25 percent equal to?
   a. 25 out of 100

b. 0.25
c. 1/4
d. all of the above
e. none of the above

32. Which of the following is the brand name for loratidine?
   a. ChlorTrimeton®
   b. Claritin®
   c. Zyrtec®
   d. Allegra®
   e. Benadryl®

33. Which category of drugs has the characteristic ending "–olol"?
   a. loop diuretics
   b. ACE inhibitors
   c. angiotensin II receptor blockers
   d. beta-blockers
   e. none of the above

34. Which of the following is an *atypical* antipsychotic?
   a. Haloperidol
   b. Fluphenazine
   c. Chlorpromazine
   d. Risperidone
   e. Loxapine

35. Considerations in determining the stability of compounded preparations include all of the following *except* which one?
   a. light sensitivity
   b. container in which the product is stored
   c. time of day when the product is prepared
   d. physical characteristics of the finished product
   e. chemical characteristics of the finished product

36. Which is the best reference to use to look up information that would appear in a manufacturer's package insert?
   a. Drug Facts and Comparisons
   b. Red Book
   c. The Physicians' Desk Reference
   d. American Drug Index
   e. Trissel's *Handbook on Injectable Drugs*

37. Which of the following is *false* regarding prescription transfer?

a. Transfer of a prescription from one pharmacy to another can be done over the phone.

b. A technician may be involved in one side of a transfer phone call as long as a pharmacist is involved on the other end of the line.

c. If no refills remain on a prescription, it may not be transferred and filled without contacting the physician.

d. Transfers are easier if the patient brings the prescription bottle to the pharmacy that will be receiving the prescription.

e. Once a prescription has been transferred, the original pharmacy must no longer refill the prescription.

38. Which abbreviation stands for "ointment"?
   a. oz
   b. OTC
   c. pr
   d. ung
   e. kg

39. Which question should be referred to a pharmacist?
   a. "Who manufactures Lovenox®?"
   b. "How much codeine is in one Tylenol #3® tablet?"
   c. "What is the difference in price between brand name Darvocet N-100® and the generic version?"
   d. "If I am allergic to penicillin, is it safe for me to take erythromycin?"
   e. "How long is the shortage of Zemuron® likely to last?"

40. Calculate the inventory turnover rate if the pharmacy's purchases for the past year were $14,845,222 and the inventory as of December 31 was $655,879 (round to the nearest whole number).
   a. 16 times
   b. 23 times
   c. 12 times
   d. 19 times
   e. 35 times

41. In which Controlled Substance Schedule does morphine belong?

   a. Schedule I
   b. Schedule II
   c. Schedule III
   d. Schedule IV
   e. Schedule V

42. All the following must be included in patient counseling according to the Omnibus Reconciliation Act of 1990 (OBRA 90) *except* which one?
   a. the name of the medication
   b. whether a generic version is available
   c. proper storage
   d. the route of administration
   e. common side effects

43. If you are to prepare an IV fluid with 2 grams of magnesium sulfate using a solution with 500 mg of magnesium sulfate per ml, how many ml do you need?
   a. 1.25 ml
   b. 2 ml
   c. 3.5 ml
   d. 4 ml
   e. 5 ml

44. Which of the following is *not* a known side effect of the tricyclic antidepressants?
   a. dry mouth
   b. constipation
   c. frequent urination
   d. blurred vision
   e. sedation

45. Which vitamin is fat-soluble?
   a. B-vitamins
   b. vitamin C
   c. vitamin D
   d. vitamin E
   e. c and d

46. Common error messages received from third-party payers include all of the following *except* which one?
   a. refill too late
   b. refill too soon
   c. invalid patient ID
   d. drug-drug interaction
   e. nonformulary, or medication not covered

47. Which of the following is true regarding the use of a laminar flow hood?
    a. Objects brought into the hood should be lined up from the back of the hood to the front to create the least turbulence.
    b. No work should be done within 6 inches from the front of the hood.
    c. Syringes should always be aimed toward the HEPA filter to avoid spraying out into the room.
    d. Objects that are not in use in the hood should be placed against either wall to keep them out of the way.
    e. The zone of turbulence around an object is roughly five times the size of the object.

48. Which is the best reference to use to look up a price?
    a. Drug Facts and Comparisons
    b. Red Book
    c. The Physicians' Desk Reference
    d. American Drug Index
    e. Trissel's *Handbook on Injectable Drugs*

49. How many 10 ml doses can be packaged from a pint of medication (round down to the nearest 10 ml increment)?
    a. 24
    b. 35
    c. 47
    d. 75
    e. 100

50. Which abbreviation stands for "four times daily"?
    a. ac
    b. qid
    c. po
    d. prn
    e. stat

51. Which of the following corresponds to "refrigerated" by USP standards?
    a. 2° to 8° C
    b. 68° to 77° F
    c. 36° to 46° F
    d. 8° to 15° C
    e. a and c

52. Which of the following are examples of automated dispensing machines?
    a. Pyxis®
    b. Omnicell®
    c. SureMed®
    d. Meditrol®
    e. all of the above

53. Which of the following is true concerning drug samples?
    a. Pharmacies may order drug samples as long as they sign an agreement not to charge patients for them.
    b. Drug samples do not require any special handling or record-keeping.
    c. It is necessary to maintain logs with receiving and dispensing information for all samples.
    d. It is acceptable to charge a small handling fee for samples to pay for the extra record-keeping that is required.
    e. none of the above

54. Which Controlled Substance Schedule denotes a drug with the least abuse potential?
    a. Schedule I
    b. Schedule II
    c. Schedule III
    d. Schedule IV
    e. Schedule V

55. Routine maintenance of the sterile compounding area should include which of the following?
    a. The laminar airflow hood pre-filter should be changed at least weekly.
    b. Cardboard should not be allowed in the area.
    c. The HEPA filter should be changed every 6 months.
    d. The laminar airflow hood should be cleaned at least every hour during use.
    e. Hood cleaning should be done from "dirty" to "clean" to avoid contamination.

56. What is 1 teaspoon equal to?
    a. ½ tablespoon
    b. 10 ml
    c. 5 ml
    d. 1/3 tablespoon
    e. c and d

57. Which of the following antihyperlipidemics is classified as a fibrate?
   a. fluvastatin
   b. nicotinic acid
   c. gemfibrozil
   d. cholestyramine
   e. none of the above

58. Which proton pump inhibitor is available as an injectable product?
   a. Omeprazole
   b. Pantoprazole
   c. Lansoprazole
   d. Rabeprazole
   e. Both b and c

59. What volume would deliver 50 mg if the solution contains 12.5 mg/ml?
   a. 2 ml
   b. 3 ml
   c. 4 ml
   d. 5 ml
   e. none of the above

60. Key areas of good compounding practices include which of the following?
   a. maintaining the compounding environment
   b. quality control
   c. ingredient selection
   d. stability of compounded preparations
   e. all of the above

61. What are Material Safety Data Sheets?
   a. sheets used by technicians to get information about hazardous chemicals
   b. sheets that contain information about how to handle a drug safely
   c. sheets that list physical and chemical properties of the drugs
   d. sheets that provide information on how to treat an exposure
   e. all of the above

62. Which abbreviation stands for "drop"?
   a. dr
   b. OD
   c. qod
   d. gtt
   e. g

63. Which question should be referred to a pharmacist?
   a. "What is the brand name of Zoloft®?"
   b. "Should amoxicillin suspension be kept in the refrigerator?"
   c. "What is the usual dose of ciprofloxacin?"
   d. "How many milliliters are in a teaspoonful?"
   e. "Is Claritin® available over the counter?"

64. Which of the following require special storage considerations?
   a. look-alike/sound-alike drugs
   b. controlled substances
   c. investigational drugs
   d. chemotherapy drugs
   e. all of the above

65. What is the *economic order quantity*?
   a. a model for calculating inventory order quantities
   b. also known as the *minimum cost quantity approach*
   c. the least amount of a drug that it is economical for the manufacturer to package for sale
   d. both a and b
   e. both a and c

66. In which Controlled Substance Schedule do the benzodiazepine drugs belong?
   a. Schedule I
   b. Schedule II
   c. Schedule III
   d. Schedule IV
   e. Schedule V

67. The Omnibus Reconciliation Act of 1990 (OBRA 90) requires which of the following?
   a. that pharmacies that receive federal reimbursement for prescriptions (Medicare/Medicaid) offer counseling to patients getting prescriptions filled
   b. that the pharmacist personally make the offer to counsel patients
   c. that all patients be counseled about their prescriptions
   d. that someone in the pharmacy counsel patients, including a technician if that person happens to be available and the pharmacist is not
   e. none of the above

68. Convert the fraction to a decimal number: 3/4
    a. 0.25
    b. 0.5
    c. 0.75
    d. 0.67
    e. 0.34

69. Which of the following is a potassium-sparing diuretic?
    a. Chlorthalidone
    b. Spironolactone
    c. Furosemide
    d. Triamterene
    e. both b and d

70. All of the following are reasons to give medications by the IV route, *except* which one?
    a. Drug characteristics make it impossible for the medication to be given by any other route.
    b. Patient is unable to take the medication by any other route.
    c. IV administration is desired for a quicker onset of action.
    d. Some medications cause pain at the injection site.
    e. all of the above

71. If you have to make 100 ml of a 10 percent w/v solution from water and a 90 percent w/v solution, how much of the 90 percent solution do you need to use?
    a. 9 ml
    b. 10 ml
    c. 11 ml
    d. 12 ml
    e. none of the above

72. Which of the following are appropriate for clean room attire?
    a. low-lint clothing
    b. no jewelry on the hands or wrists
    c. hair covers
    d. shoe covers
    e. all of the above

73. Which of the following drugs *does not* belong in Schedule II?
    a. cocaine
    b. morphine

c. propoxyphine
d. fentanyl
e. a and c

74. If you have to mix a KCl infusion with 35 mEq of KCl using a vial of KCl with 40 mEq in 20 ml, how much volume do you need to add?
    a. 3.5 ml
    b. 10 ml
    c. 12.5 ml
    d. 17.5 ml
    e. 20 ml

75. Which insulin is classified as rapid acting?
    a. Lispro®
    b. Glargine®
    c. Lente®
    d. Ultralente®
    e. NPH®

Answer Key

1. c
2. c
3. a
4. c
5. e
6. b
7. b
8. a
9. e
10. a
11. e
12. d
13. e
14. e
15. a
16. d
17. b
18. c
19. d
20. a
21. e
22. d
23. e
24. e
25. d
26. e
27. a
28. a
29. d
30. c
31. d
32. b
33. d
34. d
35. c
36. c
37. b
38. d
39. d
40. b
41. b
42. b
43. d
44. c
45. e
46. a
47. b
48. b
49. c
50. b
51. e
52. e
53. c
54. e
55. b
56. c
57. c
58. e
59. c
60. e
61. e
62. d
63. c
64. e
65. d
66. d
67. a
68. c
69. e
70. d
71. c
72. e
73. c
74. d
75. a

Index

Carisoprodol, 73
Carmustine, 74
Carrying cost, 32
Carteolol, 71
Cartrol, 71
Carvedilol, 71
Catapres, 70
CDC. *See* Centers for Disease Control and Prevention
CDER. *See* Food and Drug Administration: Center for Drug Evaluation and Research
Ceclor, 73
CeeNU, 74
Cefaclor, 73
Cefadroxil, 73
Cefazolin, 1, 73
Cefdinir, 73
Cefixime, 73
Cefotaxime, 73
Cefoxitin, 73
Cefpodoxime, 73
Cefprozil, 73
Ceftin, 73
Ceftriaxone, 73
Cefuroxime, 73
Cefzil, 73
Celebrex, 72
Celecoxib, 72
Celexa, 68
Centers for Disease Control and Prevention (CDC), 22
Centers for Medicare and Medicaid Services (CMS), 44
Centrax, 45
Cephalexin, 73
Cerebyx, 69
Cerubidine, 75
Cetirizine, 68
Chemotherapy, 11
Chibroxin, 76
Child-resistant closures, 45
Chlor-trimeton, 68
Chloral hydrate, 45
Chlorambucil, 74
Chloramphenicol, 58, 77
Chlordiazepoxide, 45, 69
Chloride, 78
Chlorothiazide, 70
Chlorpheniramine, 68
Chlorpromazine, 68
Chlorpropamide, 73
Chlorthalidone, 70
Chlorzoxazone, 73
Cholestyramine, 70
Chloral hydrate, 69
Chromium, 78
Ciloxan, 76
Cimetidine, 72
Ciprofloxacin, 18, 76, 77
Cisplatin, 74
Citalopram, 68
Cladribine, 75
Claforan, 73
Clarinex, 68
Claritin, 17, 68
Clean room, 12
Clemastine, 68
Clinical comments, 5

Clinoril, 72
Clobetasol, 78
Clomipramine, 68
Clonazepam, 45, 69
Clonidine, 18, 70
Clorazepate, 45, 69
Clotrimazole, 78
Clozapine, 69
Clozaril, 69
Cocaine, 45
Code of Federal Regulations, 46
Codeine, 45, 72
    allergy, 18
Cogentin, 70
Cold storage requirement, 28
Colesevelam, 70
Colestid, 70
Colestipol, 70
Combivent, 68
Compliance, 44-45
Compounded preparations/products, 8, 36
Compounding
    equipment, 8
    nonsterile, 48
    practice, 7-9
    processes, 8-9
    records, processes, 9
    sterile, 48
Computerized testing, 86-87
Comtan, 69
Concentration, 55
    expressed as percentage, 58-59
    expressed as ratio strength, 59
Continuous quality improvement (CQI), 44
Controlled Substance Act, 45
Controlled substances, 30, 35, 45
    ordering, 46-47
    schedules, 45-46
Copayments, 23
Copper, 78
Cordarone, 71
Coreg, 71
Corgard, 71
Cormax, 78
Cortisporin, 76
Cosmegen, 75
Cough preparations, 46
Coumadin, 71
Counseling requirements, 47
Covera HS, 71
Cozaar, 71
CQI. *See* Continuous quality improvement
Crestor, 70
Crixivan, 74
Cromolyn sodium, 67, 77
Curretab, 75
Cutosar-U, 75
Cyanocobalamine, 78
Cyclobenzaprine, 73
Cyclophosphamide, 74
Cycrin, 75
Cylert, 45
Cytarabine, 75
Cytoxan, 74

D

d4T, 74
Dacarbazine, 74, 76

Dactinomycin, 75
Dalgan, 72
Dalmane, 45, 69
Dalteparin, 71
Darvon, 45, 72
Daunorubicin, 75
DaunoXome, 75
DAW. *See* Dispense As Written
Daypro, 72
ddC, 74
ddl, 74
DEA. *See* Drug Enforcement Agency
Decimal numbers, 54
Deductibles, 23
Demadex, 70
Demerol, 45, 72
Depakene, 69
Depakote, 69
Depo-Provera, 75
DepoCyt, 75
Desenex, 78
Desipramine, 68
Desloratadine, 68
Desonide, 77
DesOwen, 77
Desoximetasone, 77
Desoxyn, 45
Desyrel, 68
Dexedrine, 45
Dextromethorphan, 68
Dextrose, 57
Dezocine, 72
Diabeta, 73
Diabinese, 73
Diagnosis, 2
Diazepam, 45, 69
Diclofenac, 72
Didanosine, 74
Didrex, 45
Diethylpropion, 45
Diethystilbestrol, 75
Diflorasone, 78
Digoxin, 71
Dilacor, 71
Dilantin, 69
Dilatrate, 71
Dilaudid, 45, 72
Diltiazem, 71
Dilutions, 59-60
Diovan, 71
Diovan HCT, 70
Diphenhydramine, 68
Diprolene, 78
Diprosone, 77
Direct purchasing, 34
Disopyramide, 71
Dispense As Written (DAW), 5
Diuril, 70
Divalproex Na, 69
Division, 54
Docetaxel, 75
Documentation, receipt of purchase order, 29, 30
Dolophine, 45
Dopamine, 18
Doral, 45, 69
Dorzolamide, 77
Dosage, 60-61
Doxacurium, 73

HIPAA. *See* Health Insurance Portability and Accountability Act
Hivid, 74
Horizontal laminar airflow hood, 12
Household measures, 56
Hydralazine, 70
Hydrea, 76
Hydrochlorothiazide, 70
Hydrocodone, 45
Hydrocortisone, 37, 77
Hydrocortisone valerate, 77
Hydrodiuril, 70
Hydromorphone, 45, 72
Hydroxyurea, 76
Hydroxyzine, 68
Hygroton, 70
Hytrin, 70
Hyzaar, 70

I

Ibuprofen, 45, 72
IBW. *See* Ideal body weight
Idamycin, 75
Idarubicin, 75
Ideal body weight (IBW), 61
Idoxuridine, 76
IDV, 74
Ifex, 74
Ifosamide, 74
IM. *See* Intramuscular
Imdur, 71
Imipramine, 68
Imitrex, 17
Incompatibilities, 10-11
Indapamide, 70
Inderal, 71
Indinavir, 74
Indocin, 72
Indomethacin, 72
Infection, 10
Infectious diseases medications, 73-76
Ingredient selection, 8
Innohep, 71
Institute for Safe Medication Practices, 2
Institutional pharmacy, billing methods, 23-24
Insulin, 73
Intal, 67
Interferon alpha 2a, 76
Interferon alpha 2b, 76
Internet, 22
Intramuscular (IM), 10
Intravenous (IV), 10
    flow rate, 61
    therapy, risks of, 10-11
Intron-A, 76
Inventory control systems, 31-33
    answer key, 41
    controlled substances, 35
    test, 40
Investigational drugs, 35-36
Invirase, 74
Iodine, 78
Ipratropium, 67
Ipratropium/albuterol, 68
Irbesartan, 71
Iron, 78
Ismo, 71

Isocarboxazid, 68
Isopropyl alcohol, 48
Isoptin SR, 71
Isordil, 71
Isosorbide dinitrate, 71
Isosorbide mononitrate, 71
Isradipine, 71
IV. *See* Intravenous

J

JAPhA. See *Journal of the American Pharmacist Association*
JCAHO. *See* Joint Commission on Accreditation of Healthcare Organizations
Joint Commission on Accreditation of Healthcare Organizations (JCAHO)
    medication management standards, 36
    policies and procedures manuals, 43
Journal of the American Pharmacist Association (JAPhA), 17
Just-in-time inventory, 32

K

Keflex, 73
Keftab, 73
Kefzol, 73
Kemadrin, 70
Keppra, 69
Ketamine, 45
Ketoconazole, 78
Ketoprofen, 72
Ketorolac, 72
Ketotifen, 76
Klonopin, 45, 69

L

Label requirements, 44
Labeling, 7
Labetolol, 71
Lactose, 37
LAH. *See* Laminar air hood
Lamictal, 69
Laminar airflow hood (LAH), 12-14, 15, 48
Lamisil AT, 78
Lamivudine, 74
Lamotrigine, 69
Lanoxin, 71
Lansoprazole, 72
Lasix, 70
Latin prefixes, 55
Legend drugs, 1
Length, 55, 56
Lente, 73
Lescol, 70
Letrozole, 75
Leukeran, 74
Leuprolide, 75
Leustatin, 75
Levalbuterol, 67
Levetiracetam, 69
Levobunolol, 77
Levocabastine, 76
Levodopa/carbidopa, 69
Levofloxacin, 76
Lexapro, 18, 68

Lexi-Comp's Drug Information Handbook, 21
Librium, 45, 69
Lidex, 77
Lidocaine, 37, 71
Lipitor, 70
Lisinopril, 71
Lisinopril/HCTZ, 70
Lispro, 73
Livostin, 76
Lodine, 72
Lodoxamide, 76
Lomustine, 74
Loniten, 70
Look-alike products, 31
Lopid, 70
Lopressor, 71
Lorabid, 73
Loracarbef, 73
Loratadine, 68
Lorazepam, 45, 69
Lorcet, 45
Losartan, 71
Losartan/HCTZ, 70
Lost order forms, 46-47
Lotanoprost, 77
Lotensin, 71
Lotrimin AF, 78
Lovastatin, 70
Lovenox, 17, 71
Loxapine, 68
Loxitane, 68
Lozol, 70
Luminal, 69
Lupron, 75
Luvox, 68

M

M-cresyl acetate, 77
Magnesium, 78
Manganese, 78
Marinol, 45
Marplan, 68
Material safety data sheet (MSDS), 22
    file, 9
Mathematical functions, 53-54
Matulane, 76
Mavik, 71
Maximizing inventory turns, 32
Maxzide, 70
Mazindol, 45
Mechlorethamine, 74
Mecloxicam, 72
Medicaid, 47
Medical devices, 37, 39
Medicare, 47
Medication administration, 85
Medication distribution
    answer key, 41
    test, 40
Medication management, 36
Medication orders, 1
    entry process, 4-5
    receiving, processing, 2, 4-5
Medications
    answer key, 81
    test, 80
Medication samples, 36
Meditrol, 33

W

Want list/book, 33
Warfarin, 17, 18, 71
Wedgwood, 9
Weight, 55, 56
    dose based on, 60
Welchol, 70
Wellbutrin, 68
Westcort, 77
Wytensin, 70

X

x-substitutions, 2
Xalatan, 77
Xanax, 45, 69
Xylocaine, 71
Xylometazoline, 77

Z

Zaditor, 76
Zafirlukast, 67
Zalcitabine, 74
Zaleplon, 69
Zanosar, 74
Zantac, 72
Zarontin, 69
Zaroxolyn, 70
ZDV, 74
Zebeta, 70, 71
Zemuron, 72
Zerit, 74
Zestoretic, 70
Zestril, 71
Zetia, 70
Ziagen, 74
Zidovudine, 74
Zileuton, 68
Zinacef, 73
Zinc, 78
Ziprasidone, 69
Zocor, 70
Zoloft, 17, 68
Zolpidem, 17
Zolpidem, 69
Zonegran, 69
Zonisamide, 69
Zyban, 68
Zyflow, 68
Zyprexa, 69
Zyrtec, 68